LESSONS

from a Golfer

A
Daughter's Story
of Opening the Heart

To Jack —
Enjoy the books

Susan C. Young

Library of Congress Catalog Card No.: 2006927226

Young, Susan Lebel
Lessons from a Golfer: A Daughter's Story about Opening the Heart
Susan Lebel Young
p. 168
1. Health—Non-Fiction. 2. Self-Personal Growth - Success.
3. Sports—Non-Fiction
1. Title.

ISBN 0-9777614-6-0

ISBN 978-0-9777614-6-3

𝒮𝒲ℬ
Just Write Books
www.jstwrite.com
Topsham, ME 04086
Printed in the United States of America

To family members everywhere:
to those whose physical hearts
open surgically
and
to those whose metaphoric hearts
open humanly
at the very same time
And to golfers and non-golfers alike:
May we all learn
the life lessons
from the links

ACKNOWLEDGMENTS

No one's heart opens alone. As the entire circulatory system of veins, arteries, capillaries, and coursing blood supports a healthy physical heart, so a network of trusted others is needed for human hearts to flourish. I am blessed with teachers who have gone before me in facing their own heartbreaks. While Dad's clogged arteries were surgically by-passed, family members helped me cut through some very old blocked places. From friends, who worked bravely with personal heartaches, I received sustenance.

Thanks, first and foremost to Mom and Dad, Jeanne and Ray Lebel. Mom's courageous walk through this labyrinth was a model for us all. And what is there to say about the man whose spirit carried us? Thank you, from the bottom of my heart, Dad, thank you. The lessons you learned on the links came through you to me when I needed them most.

To my six siblings, Mark Lebel, Ann Lebel, Mike Lebel, Vicki Lebel Koshliek, David Lebel, and Paul Lebel. We stepped into this puzzle simultaneously; we discovered the pieces together. As I worked to take the family pulse and then record it, I probably misread it often. I could not have gone through Dad's open heart surgery without you, nor would this book have ever written itself. Any mistaken understanding of your experience is mine, filtered through my limited lens. I apologize for any misrepresentation.

To my own family: Jon, husband, partner of more than a

quarter century, you support me more than you know; to Alisa, daughter, thank you for your years of twinkling eyes and radiant smiles, and for reminding me, always, of the possibility of choosing hope; to Zac, your creative wellspring flows to me and encourages me to dedicate myself to whatever passions make my heart beat.

To Paul and Anita Buckley, for the calls and visits during Dad's hospitalization, and for on-going encouragement to write.

To Roland and Janet Albert, for prompting a poem, and for the comment, "After all, families come together, don't they?"

To Paul Albert, who cared for my physical body as I paid attention elsewhere, for a much-appreciated meal at just the right time, and for being the first to call me "writer."

To Nancy Carlson, for first inviting me in the mid-1980s, to move the energy to the heart, and for continuing to stand by me with the same invitation today.

To Lisa Bussey, for reading with the pen of an editor and the heart of non-judgment, for wanting to read more, for believing in both me and the book, and for computer know-how. To Nancy DeFransesco of the Maine State Golf Association, for her editing, her journalism flair, her love of the game, and her knowing my father well enough to help me paint an accurate picture of him.

To Richard and Diane Herman, dear friends and medical professionals, for laughs, advice, comfort, and the assurance of good times even in the midst of crisis.

To my writing teachers, Michael Naylor and Joan Lee Hunter, for the constant message, "keep writing."

To Jon Kabat-Zinn, Ferris Urbanowski, Saki Santorelli, and Elana Rosenbaum at the University of Massachusetts Medical Center's Center for Mindfulness. Your first assignment for me was to "notice the openings and closings of your heart." I am still watching.

To those I dared to show early drafts of the manuscript. With heartening helpfulness, you urged me to finish. To Luis Sierra, Libby Yokum, Kaye Coker, Rebecca Stephans, Cheryl Ouellette, and Anne Ritchie, thanks for your patience and editorial comments.

To the cardiac team at Portland's Maine Medical Center, for kindness, competence, patience, and never-ending willingness and ability to answer our myriad questions. To John Love and Warren Alpern, cardiologists full of heart. And to Paul Weldner, surgeon with skilled hands.

To those of you whom I used as "golf consultants," I thank you. Mark and Vicki Koshliek, Rick Hackett, Mark Lebel, and Dad. I'm sure you tired of my endless queries. Thank you for your answers.

To Heidi and Drew Grindstaff for masterful editing, for sponsoring the book, for hanging in with me and the rewrites over the long haul. To Nancy Randolph for giving *Lessons* a name, a place, and a heart. Thank you for paying attention to the signs.

To Buffy Kay, for your heart, your expertise, your enthusiasm for this project, your friendship.

Finally, to the many unnamed friends and family members who visited, sent cards and e-mails, and made phone calls to support us. We never lost sight of the lifeline of connection, and we deeply appreciate that so many people reached out.

INTRODUCTION

OPENING THE HEART

As a man thinketh in his heart, so he is.
Proverbs 23:7

Dads are not supposed to get sick. In fact, I rarely saw my father sick. Hardly ever, as I recall, did he miss a day of work as one of Portland, Maine's first and finest oral surgeons. Never did he pass up a golf tournament. As his first daughter and oldest child, I was convinced he could do everything well. Everything. He could build dining room cabinets. He could sit in with any jazz band and play horn, with sheet music or without. He could place a tennis ball wherever he wanted on the court. He could captain a thirty-six foot sailboat. Dad just seemed to know. I was a little girl and he was a grown man: I did not think any of this was unusual. Through the eyes of an innocent child, I saw him do what I could not. It was all so very ordinary to me. Ray Lebel was simply my dad.

His hands were large for a man of small stature. At his tallest, he stood no more than five feet, seven inches tall. His hands were burly, freckled, and full of blond hair, with nimble enough fingers to trip around the keys of his trumpet, to create wonders in his woodworking shop, to wield a scalpel. He was so sure.

And he could play golf, I heard, although I was not familiar with the sport. I knew he was a champion golfer, because, when we went to the Portland Country Club for lunch now and then, I saw his name written thirty-two times on the winners' board, high on the wall on lacquered wooden plaques. He had won more club championships than anyone, ever, at any club anywhere. His club titles span seven decades. He won his first title at Martindale Country Club in Auburn, Maine in 1938, and won titles from at least five clubs since then.

I traveled with my mom to watch him play the Maine State Amateur championship every year he entered. He won that tournament six times. I learned he could play golf and I knew that he was good.

Walking from shot to shot, Dad kept to himself, and I wondered why he seemed so uninterested in socializing as he managed his game and the course. Instead of chatting as he made his way down the fairway, he did something that looked like thinking. He was not exactly thinking. He did not have a furrowed brow or that working-hard-to-understand-something kind of look. He merely focused on whatever he was doing, hole to hole all the way around, with great equanimity. On the tee, he caressed the ball in his hand and moved toward the tee, which he had placed precisely without any extra effort. Fixing his eye squarely on that little white teed-up ball as he swung effortlessly around it, he never expended any energy that was not directly related to this one thing he was doing. I heard him talk at home to my mom about "the mental game" and I figured, when I watched him, that this quiet, confident not-thinking must be part of it.

He never had a formal golf lesson. He learned golf by observing, by caddying and through his passion for the sport, becoming a student of the game. "In those days, everybody learned to play golf by caddying," he recalled. "I can't think of a healthier place for youngsters to be than out there caddying."

"Martindale is the club where I grew up," Dad admitted. Rather than hire a babysitter while they played golf, my grand-parents brought my father to the club with them. He caddied or putted on the practice green, or walked the course with them as they played their round. He won his first club championship at their course when he was fourteen years old.

He embodied something special on the golf course. Poise. Patience. Ease. Composure. I did not have words for it then, maybe not even now, but there was a sense of presence when my dad played golf. Everyone on the course felt it. His father worked for years to knock overconfidence out of him. "Pepere thought I was a cocky kid," he laughed. This quality was not cockiness, exactly. Rather he possessed an air of knowing. My dad's a winner. Maine's *Golf Magazine* in 1993, titled him "Dr. Ray Lebel of Portland Country Club, Maine's Champion of Champions." He dominated Maine Golf for most of his career.

In fact, his reputation in golf spread to the Tri-State area of Maine, New Hampshire and Vermont. He was first invited to be a member of the Tri-State Golf Team in 1940, the year he won the "Triple Crown," the Maine Interscholastic, the Maine Juniors and the Maine Amateur. His record of winning all three of those tournaments in the same year still stands. Yearly, from 1940 through and beyond 1990, he was honored to play on the Tri-State team. He reminisced, "I went to War for some of those years, but every year I was here, I played." Fifty-plus years are the longest any golfer has ever been a member of the Tri-State team. In September of 1995, the Vermont Tri-State Team awarded him a plaque which read:

RAYMOND LEBEL
Presented in recognition of his contributions
to the game of golf and to the ideals and goals pursued
and advanced by this competition,
with our gratitude, admiration and respect.

◎

Beyond the Tri-State area, in all of New England, his mastery of golf and of his own serenity were known. In 1951, he was runner-up to nationally-ranked Dick Chapman in the New England Amateur. Dad's a three-time New England Senior Amateur winner and a titleholder a dozen times in the Maine Seniors. In 1992, in the New England Seniors Tournament at the Woodlands in Newton, Mass, Dad finished his rounds, turned in his score card and was declared the likely winner. No one could beat him, the crowds believed, except maybe John Frithsen, who was still in play. Since everyone thought Dad had won, the celebration began to crown him as the New England Senior Champ. In the clubhouse, Dad waited an hour or so, and then joined the toasting. He, too, had a sip of the congratulatory champagne. Dad, staying for the presentation of "his" winners' cup, had made himself comfortable, and changed out of his spikes. His friend, Dick Marshall, offered, "I'm going back to Maine now. Do you want me to take your clubs?"

"Sure, thanks, good idea," Dad said, "take my shoes too. I'll see you next week."

He shipped his clubs, his shoes, gloves, and all golf gear home with Dick.

Then John Frithsen sank a final putt for par and tied Dad. The officials approached Dad and presented the facts. "We need a playoff," they ruled.

Emotionally centered and acting from a steady moral core, Dad nodded. With no shoes, no clubs, no glove, no gear, he agreed, "Yeah, we gotta do this. Of course, we need to have a playoff."

Dad scrounged around, borrowed a set of clubs, found someone's shoes that fit, gathered all the gear he needed, put aside his celebratory drink, and stepped up to the tee to begin the sudden death play off. John Frithsen beat him on the second playoff hole. Dad remarked time and time again as he told this story, "I didn't lose the tournament because I had a drink. I lost the tournament because John had a great shot on number two."

You see, winner or loser, Ray Lebel is a champion. Recognizing that, the executive secretary of the New England Senior Golfers' Association later wrote, "While the records will show that John Frithsen won the 1992 Jarboe Bowl in a playoff with Dr. Ray Lebel, they will not show the camaraderie and competitive spirit displayed...your response to the challenge was a display of the gentlemanly competition the game of golf fosters."

In the December, 1999–January, 2000 *Sports Illustrated* listed the magazine's choice of the top fifty greatest sports figures from each state. Raymond Lebel of Lewiston is listed as Maine's #28.

6

I never saw him sick or weak or scared, or not in charge. His heart disease hit my heart hard.

6

Warning signs of heart disease can sneak up, perhaps with sudden chest pain, shortness of breath, nausea, weakness, perspiration, or rapid pulse. Such symptoms are often difficult to perceive, because they can happen under stress and at rest, or while playing an easy round of golf. As with many people with coronary trouble, our dad did not recognize the early indicators. Tests eventually revealed that his heart suffered severe damage, from perhaps two or three heart attacks. After his cardiologist, John Love, asked if he had experienced a heart attack, Dad blurted, "No."

Regardless of our perception or non-perception, the cardiac and arterial disease process builds silently over time. As in a deteriorating golf game, the double bogeys of strokes and heart attacks can happen. Ultimately, for millions of adults, hospitalization is inevitable. In emergency rooms, urgent care begins. Nurses and doctors rush to attach monitors. Assessments by cardiac experts spew out numbers, blood test results, oxygen uptake readings, EKG tests, not unlike a diagnostic golf handicapping system. A hurried and harrying period of evaluation ensues, which at some point, breaks through our all-too-human habit of denial. With diagnoses and prognoses proposed and altered as new test results become available, patients and family alike face human vulnerability. Fear and anxiety may escalate in the person with cardiac disease and within the family. Shame, anger and guilt may also course through everyone's veins and arteries. Tighter than any narrow fairway, hospitals can smell sterile and feel cold. Even the well-visited and well-loved person can feel lonely.

And so it was for us.

Many informative books exist on the clinical aspects of heart disease and lifestyles that encourage healthy hearts. *Lessons* is different. This is the story of what happened to the emotional heart of one family in the midst of talk of ventricles and aortas. We faced tough choices. Changing events, moment-to-moment, challenged our old ways of thinking. Investigation into the occlusions and blockages in the vascular organ of one family member invited us to look into the center of our own chests.

How do we pay attention to our own heart, to what is blocked in us? How do we open our hearts when a loved one's heart is opened surgically? These are the central questions offered to you, the reader.

⑥

At some point, for every hole of golf played, the question arises, "Should I take out the pin now?" The pin is a long metal pole with a flag on the top, easily seen for hundreds of yards from the green. The pin marks where the hole is. The goal in golf is to get the little golf ball into a round sunken cup which is not much bigger than the pockmarked ball itself. That's the game. The pin is a guidepost, so the golfer can see the goal from far away and direct the shot, as skill would allow, toward the hole. Although there are no guarantees, the pin helps the golfer; it makes the outcome more predictable. After the tee shot and the fairway shots, the golfer approaches the putting green and can more accurately see the cup with the eyes; the pin can then be removed. A golfer needs to depend on his or her skill on the putting green, not on a pole, to stop the ball. Those are the Rules of Golf. Golfers can practice and learn the Rule Book, yet golf can be a frustrating game, and some days, there may be only a few good shots, no matter how many years of experience a golfer has. Generally, however, there is a pre-dictable gradual learning curve, and putts eventually get to the hole.

But for the question of how to keep the family heart open while navigating through a loved one's cardiac crisis, there is no pin. There are no Rule Books. There are no predictable out-comes, no absolute truths. No matter how much practice one has in playing the game of life, the learning curve in a hospital-ization is fast, steep and more like a roller coaster ride than a day on the driving range or the practice green. Having a loved one admitted through Emergency to a cardiac unit tests our capacity to hold tension. Through the process there are myriad questions. Answers are hard to pin down. There are only the family players trying to walk together through a medical emer-gency, as if playing golf in the high rough with no clear way through. Dad's counsel to new golfers was always to "keep it on the short grass." But we had landed in the very long brush and there was nothing smooth or easy about our path out.

⑥

Lessons is about healing hearts, at the very toughest of mo-ments, and under the scariest of conditions. This book is also about my dad, his heroism, even as those masculine hands be-came shriveled, and his forearms were shaved and grew thin. It is about his pain and joy, his times of not knowing, and how a family's collective heart helped us all—Dad included—feel less

vulnerable and alone. He learned his life lessons through golf.
Here we hear those lessons.

⑥

*The healing of my own heart began somewhere in the mid–1980s,
in a tiny building along Forest Avenue, one of Portland, Maine's
major arteries. I sat in a doctor's office. An almost-forty year old
mother of two very young toddlers, experiencing my first-ever im-
agery session, I faced a counseling psychologist. Dr. N suggested
that I needed to move energy to the heart. I had no idea what that
meant, but I was ready to try. Over the years, I had closed off my
heart to myself, and had been living with considerable self-hatred,
generated by rigid perfectionism, fueled by the need to reach unreachable standards. When the heart hardens toward itself like this,
it cannot be free to love unreservedly and to live fully. My life had
not been working very well. I had not known why, but I assumed
the therapist did, so here I was, willing. Dr. N invited me to relax,
close my eyes, envision the energy in my heart, and then describe
what I found there.*

"Are you in the heart yet?" The inquiry began.

With eyes shut, I responded, "Mm-hmmm."

"Well, what do you find?"

"An igloo."

"An igloo in the heart?"

"Mm-hmmm, an igloo." I repeated.

"How big is this igloo?"

*The thick icy walls of this isolated frozen structure almost touched
my skin. "Not very big, really...actually pretty tiny." I was beginning to feel.*

"Tell me about it."

*"It's very little, with dense blocks of solid ice. The walls are
maybe the thickness of two or three together."*

*Unaware until now that I had been scared, lonely, sad and anx-
ious, I realized in that moment that ice in the heart was going to be
the subject of our work.*

"Is anyone inside?"

"Just me, sitting alone, all wrapped up tight and small, right in the middle."

"No one else?"

"Nope."

"Is there anyone else around?"

No, there was no one anywhere to be seen. Just hard, white, vast, frozen tundra, all the way to the horizon.

"Do you want anyone else in there with you? Would you like to invite anyone in?"

"No, I don't want anyone else in here."

Now, after much softening, melting and opening, I too am a counselor. I know from personal experience, from clients in my practice, and from students in my classes, that closed hearts are everywhere. Not only are the vital organs clogged by this country's number one killer, but also the vitality in our core gets icy, a killer of different sorts. Moving from coldhearted to openhearted, as arduous as this work can be, is actually the easiest part of the journey. Staying open is the challenge, especially in the midst of inevitable ups and down. Living a path with heart asks us every moment to face our human condition without freezing up.

So it is on the golf course. It is easy to have expectations that the game will go a certain way. When it doesn't, as the twists and turns of the game plague all golfers, some people get angry, shut down, swear, and throw clubs. It is difficult to remain willing to observe, to develop post-shot acceptance, and to learn from each shot as it presents itself. In sickness and in health, on the golf course and off, when you come right down to it, the only choice we are given is to have the experience we're having. That's what golf is all about, hitting the one ball you have to hit. Not everybody plays that way.

I am coming to see that the golf my father played on the

course and off the course may not be the same as that of many of us, because he has the heart of a champion. Because he knew how to walk the links without freezing up, he played both golf and life by accepting what was right in front of him. Cursing and vulgarity grow out of thinking the game should go one way when it doesn't. Dad's golf was not the game played by club-throwers. This book tells his story, his golfer story, his human story.

⑥

I am the oldest of seven children in our large Roman Catholic French Canadian family. We are a run-of-the-mill family. We were all born in Maine and have spent our lives here. We all reside within a twenty-mile radius of Portland. We have our fun together and we have our struggles. There are sixteen years between my youngest brother and me. Two siblings are divorced; five are currently married. We are all parents; one of us has five children, and the rest have one or two. Some go to Mass regularly; others have left the Church. Three play golf; four do not. Three of us graduated from college. One of us is a vegetarian. Most of us went to public school. Mom was a homemaker. In the summer of 1998, our seven brothers and sisters organized a surprise fiftieth wedding anniversary party for Mom and Dad. The planning was filled with laughs and tearful memories, with moments of supporting each other and moments of behind-the-scenes tension. We are not the Brady Bunch.

⑥

In the summer of 1999 our seventy-six-year-old retired father underwent six-hour, seven-way by-pass surgery, in which the cardiac surgeon also repaired the mitral valve. We went through it with him. That statement is not to minimize Dad's part. His hopes and fears and experiences took him to the edge of mortality—no small matter. To underscore that loved ones go through the procedure with the patient is to highlight the fact that the family heart is called to task as well.

We had well-skilled surgeons and brilliant cardiologists in one of the top cardiac hospitals in the country. In our house, we all love our Dad. He was a first hero for many of us. Now our strong man had become a patient. The root of the word "patient" comes from the Latin, *patiens*: to suffer. Watching a patient suffer is not easy for any one.

Even as he was a patient, Dad remained my guide. He entered this surgery with the same "Yeah, we gotta do this" attitude as entering a sudden death playoff. But here the sudden death stakes were higher.

Specific family demographics and how people feel about one another may be particular in each case. Yet there is a universal: open heart surgery is emotional roller coaster material. I hope to let you, the reader, learn what this everyday family felt, thought, and did as we rolled from testing through diagnosis to surgery and beyond. With any cardiac event, the ride can be bumpy, and every possible human emotion may surface. Often clutching, sometimes screaming, now and then squealing with delight, stomachs in throats, holding a collective breath, knuckles clenched, our family tossed about.

This is not a "how to" book. Of course, there is no one right way to ride a roller coaster. What you hold in your hand is more a "how so" book, a "this is what one family experienced" documentation. Our story is surely one of many. My hope is that this map of our trip may make yours a bit smoother.

We learned that, even in difficulty, struggle, and complexity, there is a small centered place in all of us which can offer peace in the midst of life's inevitable heartbreaks and heartaches. That place is the human heart. This heart listens and speaks, gives and receives, can break open and shut down. Perhaps the healing of the world rests on separate human hearts connecting.

Dr. N. knew that individual healing depends on our becoming less vulnerable and alone. In the midst of our greatest collective crisis, the single hearts of family members pulsed. *Lessons* is about one family living through the scariest time of our lives and trying to stay aware of it as a turning point. It is about the opportunity we were given to warm up to each other rather than get cold. It is about tying up our spikes and walking the length of the course. Ultimately, it is about the opening of the human heart.

ONE

ENTERING THE UNKNOWN

Be strong then, and enter into your own body;
There you have a solid place for your feet.
Think about it carefully!
Don't go off somewhere else!
Kabir says this: just throw away
All thoughts of imaginary things
And stand firm in that which you are.
                                    Kabir

Thursday, June 17, 1999

Rushed, I slammed the back door. I was late to join my husband Jon, our sixteen-year-old son Zac, and Becca, his friend, to make our reservations for dinner in Brunswick, Maine, and then to see the Maine State Music Theater's summer production of *Joseph and the Amazing Technicolor Dreamcoat.*

The phone rang. I unlocked the door, pushed it open, grabbed the receiver which was within arm's length of the doorknob, and yelled to Jon, waiting in the car,

"I'll be right there."

"Sue, it's Mom. What are you doing now?"

"I'm flying out the door. Why? What's going on?" I asked.

Mom hesitated, "It's about Dad. I thought maybe you could......."

Her voice dropped. She rarely called and never asked for help. My heart skipped and I plopped into my kitchen chair to listen. I had an intuitive sense of what was coming. Rumblings of new fear made it hard to take a full breath and I wanted to pay close attention. "You thought maybe I could what?"

⑥

Dad had been scheduled for medical tests, so I figured this was news about the results. On Wednesday, Dad reported shortness of breath, an uncharacteristic lack of energy, lots of midday fatigue, inability to take even a few steps. As Zac and I exited my parents' home, Dad's final words were, "I am a little worried about my cardiac status."

My response at that time was a shrug of the shoulders, an inner wondering, for sure, but not alarm, definitely no sense of any danger. "H-mm," I responded, raising my eyebrows. At the moment of good-byes Wednesday night, my mind had not wandered to "imaginary things," to worst case scenarios. I assumed Dad was fine and his checkup would result in some fiddling with medication.

⑥

Mom continued. "Dad was admitted to Maine Medical Center today."

"What?" As she spoke, I looked on my wall at the 1926 color-enhanced photo of Dad at age three, building with wooden blocks decorated in alphabet letters in red, yellow and blue on each side. His grin was sly. Even as a toddler he had steady hands. I had always trusted this strength.

"Well, he drove himself to have that Doppler exam, and he

was rushed to the hospital because his blood pressure and pulse were so high. They'll do tests tomorrow. His car is there, and I wonder if you can come with me to pick it up."

When she mentioned car, a memory came.

⑥

Dad is driving, Mom sits in front, and as many kids as possible are squished into the back seat. Perhaps I am ten years old. From a very old, well-used tape, Nat King Cole is singing, "L is for the way you look at me, O is for the only one I see...." Nat King Cole has always been one of Dad's favorite singers, and Dad has played that song so much that the tape is wearing down. When there is a break in Nat's voice melody, a few bars of a clear single trumpet trill sound, and it's as if Dad is playing solo.

From the back seat, I imagine Dad playing those very same notes on his own horn. His short strong fingers tap imaginary trumpet keys on the steering wheel. During Nat's voice rests, Dad also sings Scat, "booboity, boo, buudadada. V is Very very extraordinary. E is even more than any one that you adore can love..."

Siblings feud in the back seat. "Mark touched me. Daddy, tell him to stop."

"I have to go to the bathroom, Daddy pull over."

"This is MY part. Do not go over this line. See this separation between the two seats? You can't cross over it."

"Are we there yet?"

No matter what, when the trumpet starts, Dad is the music, all the way to the end with full jazz brass jammin'. Eventually, Dad's music has a calming effect on the family and the chaos in the rear seat. He inserts the tape, drums his fingers, hums. We pause and start singing. "L is for the way you look at me..."

We all own Nat King Cole tapes today.

⑥

On the surface, anyway, nothing seemed to bother or shake

my father. I heard Nat King Cole and Dad sing at least a thousand times during my childhood, *"Love is all that I can give to you."*

As I came out of this memory, I wanted some of Dad's causal, easy way of being in the world. However, I was not sure, in this moment, just how to L O V E. Love, was indeed, all that I could give, but where and how?

©

Zac was in the driveway honking for me to hurry, pulling me out of my reverie. This was big "don't know," a huge door into the unfamiliar. Dad didn't know what was wrong. The doctors didn't know what they'd find. Mom had no idea how long she'd sleep in an empty bed. I didn't know what to do. I offered to go with her tomorrow. "Mom, how about if I go first thing in the morning with you, so I can see the play tonight?'

"I'm afraid to leave the car at Maine Med overnight."

Confusion hit. How could I leave my own family? How could I abandon my mother? Would I get to see Dad? What did they know? No longer seeing the details of my kitchen, my eyes blurred, my heart raced and my stomach tightened.

I am a typical oldest child; responsible. In that moment I was caught between two responsibilities, and I struggled with this choice. Deciding to go to the theater with my own family, I told my mother that I'd pick up Dad's car with her tomorrow. I felt the pangs of guilt building.

Mom said, "Okay. No problem, I'll get Mark to do it." I let her down, I was convinced, although she would never tell me that, and may not have even felt it. Indeed, I experienced myself letting myself down. "Should I really go? If Mom called me, she must really need help." My mind churned with internal chatter. I was scared for Dad, worried about Mom alone. Zac was still laying on the constant horn.

Mom convinced me that Mark, the next oldest, could do this. I said I'd call her tomorrow. More anxiety. "Where is my Dad? What are they doing? Will he be okay? Will Mom be able to cope? Will I be okay?"

I was disgusted after hearing how the valet parking attendant at the emergency room insisted that this weak, out-of-breath seventy-six-year-old man park his own car. I was also sad when I heard how Dad stopped four times on his walk from the car to the hospital to catch his breath. What might have happened if he had sat down? Would he ever have been able to get up? Would anyone ever find him before he died? Filled with a jumble of feelings, I was relieved that he was at Maine Medical Center, whose cardiac division is one of the best in the country, recently voted one of the nation's top 100 cardiac units. I wanted to help Mom. I wanted to offer to call my six siblings, and anyone else in our large extended family, friends. Instead I went to Brunswick, assured that Mark could do this, assured that it was too late to see Dad anyway, and assured that Mom was okay for now.

⑥

Like the beginning of every tournament Dad had ever played, we were not sure how many tricky downhill lies we would have in the upcoming bunkers. Dad was not starting this round at even par, and I sensed there may be many bogeys ahead. As a family, we were on the first tee, having had no lessons, with a club in our hands that felt wrong. There were no pros with playing tips. Thoughts, intense bodily sensations, and emotional upheaval cascaded in a torrent, all within moments of each other. Such is the nature of the mind and heart. Such was the beginning of a two-week vigil by friends and family alike.

⑥

"*Joseph and the Amazing Technicolor Dreamcoat*" is, in part, the tale of the betrayal by eleven brothers of a twelfth, Joseph. It is also the story of the importance of family, of forgiveness and reuniting. The play's themes of mercy for siblings and compassion for family were not lost on me that evening.

Nor were the challenges that lay ahead. My work over the past few years, both professionally and personally, would be needed here; that is, an ability to ride the waves of emotions and thoughts as they arise, to notice and acknowledge them, to make plenty of space for them, and nevertheless, to do what needs doing. For years, I had been teaching and learning what ancient peoples called "mindfulness." It could also be "heartfulness," as being mindful asks us to pay attention with deep reverence and acceptance to what Zorba the Greek named, "the full catastrophe" of living. When the weather is clear, skies are blue, loved ones are healthy, and moods are stable, the strong, solid, firm attitudes of mindfulness and heartfulness are tough enough.

But this day, June 17, 1999, the outside Maine summer weather as well as our inner climate had changed. With ninety-five-degree heat, high humidity, hazy skies and a father who was hospitalized for cardiac symptoms, this was certainly a time to practice what I knew, what I believed, and what was often very difficult to do:

> Keep my vision of family in mind;
> Open my heart to the feelings that arise;
> Walk through the unknown and uncomfortable, step-by-step, moment-to-moment.
> Step up to the tee, stand firm, plant the feet.

This is what I knew from my training, and from Dad's teachings. However taking "golf lessons" and playing tough courses

are two very different aspects of the game. The club was slipping in my hands.

TWO

KEEP WALKING

Keep walking, though there is no place to get to.
Don't try to see through
the distances.
That's not for
human beings.
Move
within,
But don't
move the way
fear
makes
you
move.

Rumi

Friday, June 18, 1999

This day would have been my Dad's mother's—my Memere's— ninety-ninth birthday.

Preliminary diagnosis: pneumonia. That made sense to us. Dad could not get a full breath. He was tired all the time. Many of his golfing buddies at Portland Country Club had just been treated for "walking pneumonia."

More tests were scheduled to get to the cause, to find the right treatment.

Fear planted its seeds. He was, after all, seventy-six, and had not been feeling well. The doctors and nurses were caring and competent; that was clear from the outset. His cardiologists repeated calming words to us: "Don't be concerned, we'll get to the bottom of this."

A physician's assistant tried to encourage. "Be patient, we'll figure this out."

Intellectually, we knew the truth of their intentions. We heard their words, and we believed them. Yet, when we moved within, we were not heartened.

We made phone calls. Who needed to know? Mom called Dad's usual Friday golf partners, to cancel and then we called my siblings including Vicki vacationing in California. Mark already knew. Ann was working at her new job, and her two children were at home. None of us knew how to get in touch with Mike in Hawaii. Dave arrived immediately. Paul was camping. With each call, fear moved more fiercely, as each new person contributed a story, a friend-of-a-friend tale, or a touch of personal uneasiness.

First the Maine Medical cardiac staff reported, "We do not know much for sure yet, but we do know that Dr. Lebel is a very sick man." Standing just outside his hospital room on the floor called R7, in the long sterile hall, we inhaled deeply, and exhaled a collective, "Oh, no."

Next they added, "He will probably need many more days here, and numerous tests. His condition may be serious." Hearing this, I assumed they knew more than they revealed, that they were piecing out the bad news. They were, no doubt, saving a bigger chunk for tomorrow. I was suspicious of their carefully crafted messages.

His roommate, a lanky, bearded man in the bed closest to their off-limits bathroom and to the open doorway where we gathered, spoke, "Yea, Doc, like me. I've been in here a week, and they're just now deciding what to do with me."

The nurses and cardiac doctors commented quietly to the bearded man, and then turned to us, met our eyes squarely and issued the advice, "Don't worry."

At that instant my mind blanked, because I *was* worried. I could not eat. I had not slept. I couldn't think. We muttered, "Yes, yes, of course, don't worry. That makes sense." And our terror hid underground. We did not move the way fear made us move on purpose. It was the swift and automatic response of a family taken off guard.

We were frightened, but no one admitted such a thing. We especially did not want Dad to know. We wouldn't want to worry him with our concerns. I thought that Dad was fearful too and he did not want us to know. He wouldn't want to worry us with his concerns.

I tried to remember what individual therapy, graduate school in counseling psychology, twenty years of meditation, and personal experience had taught me. I tried to remember to feel. So, when the kind and well-meaning doctors instructed me not to be afraid, I tried to listen for my own center. "Right now, what am I feeling?"

"I'm afraid," the answer reverberated. This is my Dad, my first superhero, my great teacher. This is fear." After the acknowledgment of that reality, the inner voice added acceptance: "It's okay to be frightened, Susan. In fact, it's normal."

⑥

I do not play golf. I have never had what my father calls the "yips" on the golf course. Sometimes after a round, he reported, "I had the yips. I couldn't sink a putt if my life depended on it." Often, when watching the Golf Channel, he noted a player's nervous hands, unsteady walk, inability to make the shots he wanted to make, and Dad shook his head, "Oh, the poor guy has the yips. He'll never make that putt that he needs to stay in the tournament."

If the yips dragged on for weeks, Dad had a solution: buy a new putter. As a kid, I remember counting his putters. Seventy-two at one count. New putting stroke, new putting grip, new putter. Some of these putters were four to five feet long; one hand steadies the club way at the top, the other is on the grip in the more traditional place. Some putters made ping noises; some had sight lines drawn into the club head. Some heads were huge and weighted, some thin. When Dad had the yips, he often initiated a brand new putter in a major tournament. His cronies joked, "Oh, no, Ray has another new putter."

Mom scolded, "Ray, you can't take that new putter out there for the first time today. It's a tournament. You should practice first, not take it out under major stress. "

"Sure I can," was his confident reply. "Maybe it'll break the old pattern."

I have always had the sense of what Dad meant by "having the yips," but I was never quite sure. This day I understood. My palms were sweaty, armpits wet. My own heart pounded outside my chest, my step unsure. Jittery and uncertain, I would not be able to make a decision. I had the yips.

(6

I stopped. I had worked with fear before. I knew how to feel it, and I knew I could survive it. Like Dad who eventually sank those putts, I would recover from the yips.

And so we, his family, began to move in new-putter tournament ways, ways we had never practiced before. Under the great stress of "not knowing much for sure yet," Mom made contacts all over the country, and reconnected locally, too. Some of us cleared our calendars. Others made soup for Mom. We talked to our friends, physicians, and to those who had weathered crises. We reached out to others, and reached in to our own reserves. Each in our own way, we prayed attempting to stretch beyond ourselves.

❦

I e-mailed friends who had never met Dad and they sent back well-wishes. I sat at my computer, looking out my den window at the summer blues and greens, eyes glazed over. The outside heat and my inner fog blurred the colors. At the end of my driveway, my young friend and neighbor, three-year-old Sammy Malone screamed, "Come on, Daddy, push me on my Big Wheels." A memory surfaced of my own father, running behind my new two-wheeler, pushing on that little black seat, letting me go at just the right moment. Memories cascaded of a more youthful, healthier Daddy.

My fingers flew frantically across the computer keyboard, recording whatever spilled out the ends of them, through the keys and onto the screen. I was clearly not thinking. I did not dare to open the circuits in my mind which could so easily spin worst case scenarios. No, this was not thinking, and the typing was so rhythmic and automatic that it numbed all emotion. I was so filled with the yips that the hope in my fingertips was that I was writing fiction. The truth poured onto the screen, but I did not want to believe it.

We all had our feelings in this family and we kept walking. We picked up our new putters, we tried to break old patterns of panic and fear and we initiated our brand new skills under major stress.

THREE

PAUSING

One very simple tip will definitely improve the timing of most golfers. Merely pause briefly at the top of the backswing.
Tommy Armour

Saturday, June 19, 1999

Pause we did: Congestive heart failure. My own heart quickened when I heard today's diagnosis. I knew nothing about this condition medically, but I had witnessed its toll on patients and family alike. I remembered a family who had also visited this floor several times during my year as a pastoral student here. Howard Lynn, (names have been changed), the father in the family, was living with congestive heart failure. Simultaneously, he was dying of it. Having counseled Howard and his wife Clara on each of his several admissions, I paused at the top of this backswing, this flashback. I remembered how his lungs filled with fluid, just as my dad's had last week. I remembered his labored breathing, sounding like my dad's. Every few weeks, Howard arrived at the hospital in crisis, became stable, left with a new medication regime, and returned several weeks later, more severe each time. His heart could no longer pump to extremities. His feet became shiny and bluish, hands clammy. He eventually made the decision not to be a hospital patient. He wanted to die at home. For a month or so, hospice workers ushered Howard and Clara through his final days. Invited by Clara a day before Howard left this world, I visited their loving home, and prayed with the Lynns. Surrounded by his daughters and wife, Howard's was a beautiful death; a death nonetheless. Thoughts of the past scared me.

Congestive heart failure. Pause. My dad never met the Lynns, nor the other families with similar experiences. Although he had not heard my stories of working on these cardiac floors five years ago, he, too, remembered the past. His mother died of congestive heart failure when she was only a few years older than Dad was then. Dad had watched his beautiful mother fill with fluid, until she was hardly recognizable. What must he be thinking now, so close to her birthday, hearing this same diagnosis? I asked him. He was quiet, reserved. His only comment was, "I wish I had paid more attention to the cardiac information at Tufts Dental School."

Wondering how that past might be affecting him now haunted me. Dad mentioned, too, that his dad, his uncle and his aunt, indeed much of his family, died of heart disease. Focusing on the past was clearly not steadying.

What about the future? I called my dear friend, Richard, a family doctor, to ask about the prognosis for congestive heart failure. "Well, he'll eventually die of it, but he can live some years, pretty comfortably 'til the end."

6

In this dangling moment of not knowing what the future held at the Maine Medical Center in Portland, Maine, Dad shared with me his attitude. He had no idea how helpful his wisdom was: "I am so grateful to be at the Maine Medical Center, because I know it has a great reputation for cardiac care." Pushing with his palms, he shifted in bed, wincing as he propped himself up.

"These young doctors are really smart. They made the decision to come to Maine consciously—to live well. They're good people as well as competent physicians." This is the spirit I had come to love.

"The nurses are incredible. Everyone is so helpful here and has all the right information." Now the sunshine caught his narrow gray-green eyes, and there was a spark in them that I recognized as what he calls "the zone."

⑥

In golf, he has always told us, "When you're out of the zone, it means you're not concentrating. The mind can go toward the negative. Then you can't get it done. How you think is really important, because if you're not a positive thinker, you can visualize the trajectory of the shot all you want, you can know how far you want it to go, and none of that will matter. You won't be able to make anything happen. The zone is a way of concentrating, a way of having proper confidence in what will happen. It's like you can talk yourself into what you want to do. It's not really about thinking. It's about being in the zone. It's hard to describe in words."

⑥

In the zone now, he talked himself into proper confidence, perhaps even a positive trajectory for his care. "I am so glad to be home in Maine rather than in Florida. Just imagine if this had happened there last winter. I wouldn't have all the kids around, or all these friends." The gratitude of the identified sick person, his presence, steadied me, gave me—this able-bodied one who could walk out of this hospital—pause.

He added, "You know, Jack Nicklaus once said, 'Golf is not

and never has been a fair game.' That's just like life. Sure, I wish I weren't here, in one way, of course, but if I have to be in this situation, worrying about its fairness won't help. I just want to do what needs doing, and I'm happy to be here to do it."

I asked him once if he thought he was born with this ability to stay calm and one-pointed, or whether he learned it in his various roles. Did he choose what he wanted to do because of this talent he has to be steady in the midst of a storm? Did his gifts come first and then his path? Or did he develop his great abilities because of his life situations? When I finished asking, he looked blankly at me and answered, "I don't know what you're talking about."

Dad did not think as much as I do. As a World War II Navy fighter pilot in the South Pacific, he faced his flight every day, uncertain whether he would return. Fearlessness is not the same as having no fear. Rather, it has more to do with courage, and he had that same courage now in this uncomfortable, confused pause. Indeed, the word courage comes from the French word for heart, *coeur*. It was his mechanical heart in question, but I never doubted that his metaphoric heart was still perfectly healthy, alive and well.

I remember a story he told of being in the middle of the Pacific on an aircraft carrier during the holidays. Someone thought it would be a good idea to play Bing Crosby's *I'm Dreaming of a White Christmas*. Dad recalled, "Every soldier on the ship was in tears."

It was this heart I trusted—this tender heart which buoyed me in this moment. Physically, Dad was withering; lost six pounds in one day from the diuretic. His wedding ring swam around his finger. Even as I witnessed this shriveling, the memory of that picture he showed us so many times comes to me; the one of him young, strong, brave, handsome, muscular, in his Navy whites, holding the Distinguished Flying Cross awarded to him for shooting down two enemy planes in one mission.

I also asked Dad once if he learned this ability to stabilize in an emergency through his training as a surgeon, with his attention needing to be solely on the surgical field. Again, he had no answer.

As a young girl I wondered, "Daddy, do you get nervous paying golf with so many people watching you?"

"No."

"Really?"

"Well, if I let the pressure get to me, I wouldn't be focused where I need to focus. Golf is a mental game."

He has always understood naturally what many of us struggle to learn; presence. "When I hit a golf ball, I only hit this golf ball right in front of me. If I am still stewing about the last shot I hit, or worried about the upcoming putt, it can only hurt me. Golf is one stroke at a time. The only important question is 'what kind of lie do I have right here?' The lie of the ball is the position of the ball relative to how easy or how difficult it is to play. Sometimes you get a good lie; sometimes you get a bad lie. The degree of difficulty doesn't really matter. Sometimes you get lucky, but always you get what you get, and the game of golf is to hit that little ball from the tee to the hole."

⑥

I am not a golfer, but I listen for wisdom. Dad taught me to stay balanced in the midst of ups and downs, gains and losses, victories and defeats. In order to be open to what might be possible, he suggested that I practice calm-centeredness in the present moment. Otherwise, I might have been paying attention to my busy mind thinking upsetting thoughts, or to my feelings creating more turbulence, or to the noisy halls of the hospital, the parade of roommates, and the mounting diagnostic evidence of a very sick heart.

The lie of Dad's past unwanted golf shot held both challenge and opportunity. So, too, did this crisis. As the family ruminated on what was "wrong," Dad, with his sanity and wisdom, clued us in that this "present" also offered great gifts. How we experience this life is a matter of where we place attention—a matter of perspective.

"You never know what these bright young doctors and their new modern medicine can do. I don't know much about this, but these guys are wonderful. This cardiac team is great. This is all very promising."

With those words, it's as if he had just played a provisional ball. When in doubt, pause, play safe, have another plan, and leave yourself plenty of opening for new possibilities.

FOUR

LISTENING WITH THE EARS OF THE HEART

. . .music heard so deeply
That it is not heard at all, but you are the music
While the music lasts.
T. S. Eliot

Sunday, June 20, 1999 ✎ *Father's Day*

"Why?" My good friend Diane, a nurse, asked me. "What's causing the congestive heart failure?"

Good question. The doctors wondered, too. More tests.

I called Diane, as I had many days, to connect with a "medical expert," to run the latest findings by her scientific knowledge, and mostly to reach out to a confidante.

"Cardiomyopathy."

An extended silence gaped on the other end of the phone. Diane's voice deepened. "Oh….."

She stopped. I was speechless. This was not instant reassurance. Unformed words caught in my lumpy throat. I couldn't articulate the dread pounding in the middle of my chest. Only vaguely did I sense my mind falling into a dark pit.

Diane's voice lowered yet again. "That's not good."

@

I knew even less about cardiomyopathy than congestive heart failure. Images swirled of "failure," or of lungs "congesting" with fluid, and Dad, forced to take diuretics then peeing away pounds of weight merely to be able to breathe. And cardiomyopathy? That the heart has trouble pumping blood. That this can lead to heart failure. I recalled that one of these conditions, in younger people, is treated with a heart transplant. Clearly not good.

My fathers's past gave little indication of any of this. He had a strong constitution, solid will, was actually a youthful seventy-six. Yet the future was looking more and more grim. Dave groaned, "Every time we hear an update, it's scarier than the last. The news has all been bad news, and it goes from bad to worse."

The human heart is a non-rational, extremely sensitive receiver. This was a time not only for medical analytical understanding. Something more was happening here; my heart was stirring.

The words of French philosopher, Blaise Pascal, rang out, *"The heart has its reasons that reason will never know."*

For reasons that reason could not explain, I gave up hope.

@

This was a good thing. Letting go of hope released all future expectations. I came to believe that this moment was all I had, was all Dad had. "This Father's Day is it." This was not a Father's Day like many others, when he played the Father/Son Tournament, which later included also the Father/Daughter, and had been renamed the Parent/Child Tournament at the Portland Country Club. It was always his favorite place to be on Father's Day, battling it out with the other big families who had been his great friends and rivals for years: Pierce, Blais, Noyes, Franceour. This was a Selected Drive Alternate Shot Tournament; both players hit a tee shot, and then chose which to use to continue. The players alternated shot-by-shot until the last putt of each hole, and started each hole again with two tee shots.

Once Pepere, Dad, Mark and Mark, Jr. all entered. Dad and Mark signed in as both a father and a son. This led to much hilarity. Dad hit two balls off the tee, one of his as the son of his own father, who had hit one; and one as a dad. Mark hit the other shot as a son, and also hit a second shot as a father, for his son Mark, Jr. to play, too. Dad hit two balls, and Mark hit two balls, while Pepere and Mark Jr. each hit one, all the way around on every tee. So as not to confuse balls, they color-coded each ball with magic marker to keep track. "It was comical. We had a great match, four generations out there," Dad remembered, and added, "By then end, we felt as if we had each played a thousand holes of golf."

Mark and Dad had played this Parent/Child Father's Day tournament at least fifteen years, and won it "a bunch of times." Mark remembered one tournament when he was thirteen or fourteen years old. On number five, Dad hit a really beautiful drive, almost to the green. All Mark had to do was hit a short wedge, maybe run it up close to the pin, so Dad could putt for a three. Mark took his back swing, and shanked it. The ball skipped over the trees, over some out-of-play dirt, over a fence and sank to the very bottom of the Portland Country Club swimming pool. PLOP! It plummeted into the water. Mark laughed, "Dad is so patient, always so calm out there. He never gets rattled, or at least he never shows it. He's always positive. He calmly took a ball out of his bag and, without expression, simply stated the rule. 'Okay, we have to hit another one.'"

Dad dropped a new ball, hit a wedge to the green and then it was Mark's putt. Dad relaxed the whole time. Because Dad had always practiced letting go of any hope of things being different than they were, he was free to hit his one shot, unencumbered by thoughts of what might be next. This ability to accept reality— as it is— has never changed in him, on the course and off. He became equanimity.

This Father's Day, Dad did not enter the Parent/Child tournament, but there was plenty of Parent/Child, Child/Parent love just the same. Dad was unrattled; at least he was not showing it. Patient and calm, he rested comfortably. With cardiomyopathy as a diagnosis, I was not so positive as Dad. Who knew what would be next? I felt sunken to the very bottom of the deepest water hole.

I told Dad years ago I was not then interested in golf, that, "maybe when I'm eighty, I'll take up the game."

"It'll take you that long to learn how to play," he teased.

Indeed, golf professional Gary Player quipped, "Golf is a puzzle without an answer. I've played the game for forty years and I still haven't the slightest idea how to play." In this moment of dropping all hope for a future cure, the tension I had carried on my breast bone softened, my shoulders fell back into their sockets from their temporary spot next to my ears, and my chest relaxed, in an embodied admission that I did not have the slightest idea how to play this game of life, which I'd been at for over fifty years. When I abandoned hope, the holding loosened, the grasping fingers opened, the tight jaw slackened, and the wishing ceased. I felt free.

Webster's Encyclopedic Dictionary defines "cure" as: "successful remedial treatment; to relieve or rid of something troublesome or detrimental; restoration to health." Curing is not always possible, and it looked more and more unlikely for Dad. Healing is different. That same dictionary defines "heal" as: "to make whole or sound; to cleanse, to purify." The word "heal," derives from the same source as the words holy, healthy, and whole. Healing is always possible

I brainstormed Father's Day gift ideas that would help Dad feel whole, something healing. "When is he the happiest? On the golf course. Not possible now and he has spent the last weekend on this cardiac floor enjoying peace and solitude watching the *U. S. Open* on his wall-mounted hospital TV. This was enough for him, another example of his innate ability to make the best of things."

A golf theme did not ring true for me as a healing tool. It might only trigger sadness in him, I imagined, regret at not being on the course. I wanted this Father's Day present to sing to me, to sing to him.

"What else does he love? How would he choose to spend his last days? (which-I-can't-tell-him-I-imagine-to-be-his-last-moments-and-I-wonder-if-he-thinks-these-are-his-last-moments-too-and-he-doesn't-want-to-tell-me-so-I-can't-ask-him-for-his-preferences-so-I'll-have–to-read-his-mind-and-hope-he-isn't-reading–mine)"

✿

Music. Dad was a jazz trumpet player; a big band musician at heart. His dad, a man who had made his living playing horn for a time, was his teacher. My father's music evoked relationship with his dad, and he passed on the legacy; we all took music lessons. Jazz had been an outward inter-generational link, and it also connected him inwardly to a huge part of himself. Like the Parent/Child Tournament he played with his own dad, his son and his grandson, music equaled family. From the time he was a toddler, that trumpet had coursed through his veins, and had been associated for him with kin, fun, creativity, letting loose, enjoying technique, and appreciating stirring sounds and creative musicians.

Dad played in bands to help pay for his schooling at Bowdoin College, in Brunswick, Maine. We grew up with the sounds of Louis Armstrong, Ella Fitzgerald, and Sarah Vaughan. Even after years of not practicing, even after not remembering how to read music, Dad could and did become his horn every time he lifted it to his lips. He stood in with swing bands, dance bands, any band that would ask him—and many did.

One of my favorite photos of Dad shows him at my wedding in 1975, dressed in his father-of-the-bride tux, blowing his brass instrument: hands, arms, shoulders in perfect position; head leaning back; lips pursed; eyes shut; soul shining through. That photo embodies Dad's spirit, connects me to my childhood, to hearing Dad play; to his dad and the two of them playing together; to Dad's childhood playing horn, and perhaps even to his dad's childhood and music. That jazz trumpet is happiness for me: for Dad too.

ⓖ

As a teacher and student of mind-body approaches to wellness, and as a meditation instructor, I was cognizant of the studies which show that, for some of us, music is more pleasurable than any other activity. Research documents the release of endorphins when we hear music we love. These "feel good" hormones relieve pain and induce states of bliss. There is evidence that certain kinds of music for certain people have the same effect as low doses of Valium. Music can reduce stress. It can make us feel younger. The field of music therapy helps treat depression, and medical problems such as cancer, stroke, arthritis, diabetes, headaches, and more.

ⓖ

But it was not science that led me to buy Dad a Discman and a few choice CDs. Connecting with the trumpet was to help heal his heart—not cure, not the circulatory pump. I imagined flow of a different kind; the awakening of life force energy. The human heart is more than the mechanical pump which sustains physical life. It is a listening apparatus. "True musicians do not listen to music with ears alone," my pianist friend Rebecca reminded me. "They listen with the heart."

If Dad could hear and become his music, healing would begin, I imagined, tears would flow, and laughter would erupt. My idea for buying this particular Father's Day gift, then, sprang from what I knew about him as a man. My decision to hunt down Louis Armstrong and Nat King Cole was less about killing endless hospital hours, and more about enjoying each moment. After all, we were being shown through this crises that time is not endless. It is precious.

I shopped, wrapped, delivered the package to him. Sleeping on his left side when I arrived, he wore a clean white Johnny. Stirring a bit when he sensed someone, his eyes opened to slits, "Oh, hi Sue," he mumbled.

"Happy Father's Day," I greeted him with a forehead kiss.

With raw elbows from the bed sheets, his shaking hands opened the little gray-wrapped box. When a look of surprise and delight enlivened him, tears welled up and collected in my eye sockets, but I did not let them fall. "Oh, I love Satchmo." His words commingled with the synchronized movement of his donning the earphones and beginning the finger tap.

The music he heard in his new headset was, in fact, transforming. He cried with Louis' words. I cried, too. Nat King Cole comforted us. Spontaneous memories emerged: trumpet lessons with his dad; songs he struggled to learn to play. Tears streamed down his cheeks as he recalled, "Oh, it's 'Basin Street Blues.' I love this song. It's really an oldie, one of his early ones. I wanted to play 'Basin St. Blues' for so long as a kid and I kept asking my father if I could learn it. I begged him to teach it to me, or get me the sheet music. Pepere insisted, 'No, you're not ready to play that song. Go back to your scales.' I thought I was ready long before he did, and when I finally got to practice this music, I was so happy. I love this song."

He reminisced about other beloved songs. His face softened. A type of casual, informal life review unfolded as he listened: here a memory, there a story, now an old joke. For me, this day, the well of hope was empty. I imagined his black trumpet case gathering dust, and the next party without hearing his horn. If Dad's music would be silenced for future Father's Days, at least he could be fully present in this moment, resting with a grin, tapping his fingers and toes. That's healing.

@

There's an old joke that a well-adjusted man is one who can play golf as if it were a game. Dad persevered, with unshakable courage, facing higher-level doubts and fears than those dog-legs to the left, the wide bunkers, the deep water hazards, and the pins at the back of the green. One plays golf, one plays music, and this well-adjusted man played the edge of life with hot cheeks, warm tears and laughter.

FIVE

FEELING EMOTIONS

The heart is
The thousand-stringed instrument.
Our sadness and fear come from being
Out of tune with love.

Hafiz, the great Sufi master

Monday, June 21, 1999

"Mom, hi, how are you today?" This was the first phone call I made each morning. Dad lay in the hospital receiving competent care. Daily, Mom returned home alone.

"Oh, Sue, today is the first day I've felt..." her voice trailed.

She choked, unable go on. My mother is no more than 5'4" with beautifully thin legs, a head small enough so that hats never fit. Her long fingers, with manicured nails, could be models for the diamond rings she wears so loosely. Her feet are so narrow that she needs AA or AAA width shoes. Slender by nature, she is nevertheless tough, articulate and, taking after her own mother, the kind of small woman you would want on your side.

She fought the local school board when she felt the town had not given one of her sons a fair shot in school. With straight white teeth, highlighted hair, a picturesque smile, and a flair for conservative, Talbot's-like fashion, she is mostly what you would call a lady. A lady with a stiff upper lip. She tells stories of being ridiculed as a child when she cried. She tells stories of going toward her dad to kiss him goodnight and getting the feeling that she was being a "sissy."

This day she was crying, just a little. I could feel her upper lip trembling, wavering ever so slightly. No doubt she was holding back, so as not to appear weak.

In our family, we never talked much about feelings. Emotions were "silly," or perhaps more accurately, a bother in a busy household. Dad was stoic on the golf course, quietly walking. After his own great shots, or after a partner's, which might land right in the middle of the generous fairway, he simply acknowledged it with an even-keeled, "Nice play."

And, if his putt from the fringe rolled right up to the hole, caught the lip of the cup, rimmed around it a few times, then dropped in for a spectacular birdie, he smiled a bit. "Yes," he'd bob his head, pick up his ball, and amble to the next tee. When he hit the ball in the woods, which was rare, he took a deep breath, and just as silently, kept the play moving.

No, we had not been demonstrative with emotion in our family. This was a tough time to learn.

"Scared?" I asked Mom, "disheartened?"

Silence. Again, no words, although I had the sense she was nodding her head, biting her lip, squinting her eyes. "Mmmm."

I heard her sniffling. I heard her fighting back tears.

"Sad?"

"Yeah."

"Lonely?" Surely the possibility of losing her husband of fifty-one years was a complex web of emotion.

"Mmm-hmmm."

"Me, too." I joined her. We were together in this as family, as human beings.

"Okay." We agreed.

We breathed together, a sigh of connected relief. She inhaled and exhaled without the crutch of a cigarette. Perhaps she would light up after this early morning check-in. For now, we simply hung together in this suspended moment, this big extended now. I waited on the other end of the phone, but we were done talking. There was nothing else to do, nowhere to go, although my mind struggled to be still.

⑥

Emotions are normal, natural, though often difficult. So, because tight stomachs, closed throats, light-headedness and heaviness in the heart are so unwanted, we fear getting thrown off the track of the roller coaster. Believing that we won't survive, we work hard not to feel the unpleasantness. All seven of us had been walking the line between consolation, cheering up, and trying to forget the internal upheaval. The siblings stayed close. David invited Mom to his house for a lobster dinner. Mom was thankful; they laughed and distracted themselves for a while. Later that same evening, Mark called to see how Mom was doing. As I would the next morning, he sensed her welling up with emotion. Mark told her he'd be right over and they could have a drink together, which would help her sleep. She appreciated his visit, his thoughtfulness, and a good night's rest. Ann, also breaking down, offered to spend the night with Mom. Grateful for the offer, Mom nevertheless declined, "No, no, I'll be "Okay."

Calling from her vacation spot in California, Vicki heard daily updates and offered support. Paul dropped by to see if Mom needed help with anything. Mike was still unreachable. I made the morning phone call, met Mom for lunch, and drove to the Medical Center with her.

This family was together in this most common human experience: emotion. Being in close contact with each other, and with Mom, was comforting. Relationships are, in fact, crucial, especially in crisis. Yet, even with our best efforts to soothe, to stay in tune with love, we were nonetheless frightened and confused. Most of us had not learned how to embrace and work with all this internal chaos. Outwardly, we grew in connection as a family. Inwardly, we were left alone with our individual terror and dread, and our not knowing what to do.

How do we learn to experience emotion, to feel, when our conditioning taught us differently? After all, many of us remember growing up with contradictory puzzling messages. When we had trembling inside, or lumps in our throats, we looked to adults—in churches, in schools, at home, on the playing field— for help dealing with this discomfort. They had no training either.

⑥

This day we waited. More tests. More work to determine the underlying cause and nature of Dad's diseased heart. Through all the diagnostic studies, a picture began to emerge of a severely limited heart muscle, working at only twenty percent of its capacity: no life in the left ventricle. Suspicion built that Dad's congestive failure may not have been the primary pathological process. A thalium test showed limited blood flow to the heart muscle. Coronary artery blockage needed be investigated. We heard the first talk of coronary by-pass surgery.

What are my emotions?

Fear?
Mmmm.
Sadness?
Yeah.
Loneliness?
Mmm-hmmm.
Okay.

There was no fixing. There were no definitive answers. There was only supporting each other, only love. There was only feeling, of course, and patience. As a kid I was too fidgety to play golf. Perhaps I was too young when I started, or too vigorous. I could never still my inner busyness. It was the same at MMC. Restless, aching to run. Anxious energy whirling. A tug to hurry up. All these feelings rushed at me. I did not know what to do with them.

Dad knew. Before he left the house for the finals of the Maine State Amateur Championship one year, I asked him, "Dad, you seem so unruffled when you play golf. How do you stay calm on the course? Don't you get scared? Don't you get angry when your opponents throw their clubs? Don't you get mad at yourself when you make a bad shot?"

His answer came easily, not through introspection. It is rather by his life experience, and through his actions, that he has always explained his life lessons, his philosophy. "What my opponents do is beyond my control. I only have control over my own game. The fact that my last shot was not what I wanted is in the past already. Of course I have feelings on the course. Everyone has feelings. By the time I walk up to the ball, I simply have to do what needs doing. If I want to win—and if I enter a tournament, I DO want to win—I have to notice and accept those feelings so they don't rule my game. Then I have to walk up to the ball and hit the next shot. You know, my opponents always say, 'Ray, you're so calm. You never show any emotion.' And they're right. I never show any emotion on the outside, but I always tell 'em they have no idea what's going on inside me. Sometimes inside I'm all worked up, but I don't want to show it to them. That emotional curve is a horrible curve. It can get too high on a good shot and too low on a terrible shot, and I want to stay at an even emotional level. So I stay patient on the outside, keep my cool, which helps the inside stay calmer too. I meet the good and the bad shots all the same, with the same emotion, which is no emotion on the surface. There's a lot of waiting in golf—on the tee while others are hitting, on the fairway while others take their shots, walking to your next shot, and on the putting green—and it is in those waiting moments when the mental game kicks in. I can't let my feelings boss me around. Sure, feelings come and go, and, through it all, I keep playing the game."

(6

And so I felt the terror and the uncertainty in me on the inside, but I did not show it to him. I kept playing the waiting game.

SIX

CHOICE-MAKING

Be patient toward all that is unsolved in your heart
And try to love the questions themselves.
                              Rainer Maria Rilke,
                              Letters to a Young Poet

Tuesday, June 22, 1999

Yearly, we looked forward to this day in my family. Sixteen-year-old Zac was leaving for summer camp. No longer was he the chubby preadolescent who wore only oversized sage green t-shirts and forest green Umbro shorts with Birkenstocks, never any socks. No longer did he sleep the whole six-hour ride from Portland, Maine to the Catskills in New York, or slump in the back of the car with this headset on, singing above his *Miss Saigon* CD. Now he was proud of his bright, straight white teeth, his shaven chiseled chin, his broad shoulders and trim waist, and he was awake much of the way looking in the mirror. "Vanity check," we teased when we caught him, and he laughed at our jokes now that he was on the upper end of the teenage years.

He would be pleasant in the car.

For two weeks now, we had been buying Arm and Hammer Advanced Whitening Dental Care toothpaste, Degree Shower Clean deodorant in the green tube, and stage makeup. This was theater camp, his favorite place. Writing his name with a black Sharpie laundry pen on his boxers, on his green flannel sheets, on the arches of his socks, we spent evenings reminiscing of past years. Excited to reconnect with his old camp friends, Zac's e-mail activity and long-distance phone calls had been increasing. Zac was eager for Jon and me to meet his theater buddies again. In the car we sang Broadway show tunes to Zac's many CDs. He had the complete soundtrack of *Rent* planned for us today. We would take breaks at special, well-visited stopping places along Massachusetts' Route 495, and Connecticut's Route 84.

Jon and I had also been looking forward to the return ride as uninterrupted moments of "married time." Each trip, we'd talk. We'd catch up. I learned things about his life and his work that, even though we had lived together for more than a quarter century, I had never before heard. As wonderful as this verbal bonding was, we also enjoyed long stretches of silence, in comfort, just being together. Of course, we, too, had our favorite eating spots.

In particular, I looked forward to this day for me, as I had spent the last week juggling counseling schedules, trying to be in many places at the same time. Work. Write to Zac's sister, Alisa, who was away for the summer. Visit Dad. Be with Mom. Get Zac ready. The upcoming twelve hours in the car would allow me to sit still, meditate some while Jon drove, and belt out tunes when I would take the wheel and Jon would sleep. Scheduling no clients today, I was free to go. The day was mine; for my family and for me.

But I was twitchy. Today Dad was scheduled for a cardiac catheterization. The results of this minor diagnostic surgery would let the doctors know if there was coronary artery blockage, and, if so, the severity. A tube would be placed in his femoral artery, a dye then injected and its path to the heart monitored. For six hours after the procedure, Dad's leg would be immobilized, kept absolutely still, in order to prevent hemorrhaging. He would be sedated during the exam, and for the hours after. Dad would be out of his room much of the day, and slightly out of consciousness for the rest of it. Daily visits to Dad had become routine for me. I liked them. Today would be the same, except that he may not even know I was there.

It was not the logic of the details that caused my uneasiness, my questioning. As I felt yanked in one direction to go to New York with Zac and Jon, my heart jerked me the other way, too— to find a way to be with my Dad. Can I visit Dad before I leave for New York at 6 a.m.? Or after the return at 9 p.m.? The first time I turned my attention to my heart several years ago, I found an igloo. This day, I was listening to my heart and there waged a tug-of-war.

Tug.

Pull.

Push.

Ask.

Question.

Painful dilemma. The possibilities were at war with each other; my heart was the battlefield. Fear arose that Jon might be feeling neglected this past week, that he might be angry or disappointed if I chose to stay in Maine. Convinced that these were Dad's last days, I wanted to eke out final moments with him. I wanted to be with Mom, on this, the toughest of days yet. This was final evaluation day.

Caught in the sandwich generation, I wrestled with self-doubt. The questions were tough, but it began to occur to me that I did, indeed, have choices. Starting to entertain the idea of hugging Zac and Jon early, I hesitated, as if I needed their sanction.

Zac bounced up and down the stairs in his skin-hugging black t-shirt, muscular arms doing the work of lugging boxes and crates from his second floor apple-red bedroom. Crashing down the green carpeted stairs, through the dining room, then through the kitchen, finally tripping over fans and suitcases in the mudroom, Zac let the broken screen door slam behind him. He headed one last time out the back door to finish loading the Jeep in the driveway. He had showered, as his "Phantom of the Opera Eau de Toilette" announced. I could tell he was almost ready to leave by the newly donned designer jeans. I knew when he was close by the whiff of citrus "Fudge Oomf Booster," which he scrunched into his close-cropped brown-black hair. He was 5'5, more a man now than my little boy. His deep, resonant, classically trained tenor voice was belting a song from the musical, *Pippin*, "I Am What I Am."

On one of these last trips through the kitchen, I stopped him. Sheepishly, I bumbled, "Zac, I was thinking…um…how would you feel about it if…ah…what would you think if I…I mean…I really want to go to camp with you, but…like…maybe I'd rather…you know…I have this feeling I should be with Memere and Pepere."

Aaauughh. There I got it out. Waiting for his temper tantrum, or pout, or tirade of guilt-producing screams, I held my breath.

Through his deep-set brown eyes, Zac gazed at me with ultimate ease and nonchalance. His voice calm, soft, he answered, "Well, Ma, if you're looking for my permission, I don't really care. I can do a lot of the driving on the way out, so Dad can rest before he heads home. It actually makes sense to me that you stay here."

Phew. One hurdle. Tension released a bit in my jaw and shoulders. Zac was growing up, maturing. He was healthy, happy, and responsible. I saw it, sensed it. His smile was wider, his face more open, his shoulders broader rather than stooped. My heart softened as appreciation welled for Zac's compassion and understanding. I was proud to be his Mom.

Then I felt tingly again, afraid to ask Jon. Why? I didn't know. Jon is kind, gentle, generous, and reasonable. His teddy-bear build and cuddly tummy are as cozy as his voice is clear and soft. When confronted with internal or external conflict, he strokes his red moustache, running his freckled fingers over his upper lip and down his shaven chin again and again. He closes his green-gray eyes, goes inside. Then he relaxes with a "hmmmm." Jon's five foot, eight inch frame softens under duress; silence is his default position.

But this day's spot on the roller coaster had already delivered many feelings: anticipation, doubt, fatigue, discomfort, love, confusion, gratitude, softening, pride, fear. It was not yet 6 a.m. Now here was insecurity, a feeling of not having "been here" much for Jon lately. Maybe he'd hear my question as "I don't want to be with you." The human mind tosses about so.

"Jon......I already talked to Zac and......I mean......well....so I was sort of thinking.....you know?........Um......like... I assume, kind of... that Mom is going to be alone all day today......like, you know, I figured I could......maybe......if it's okay with you.......stay'n'be-with-her."

............Pause.......Jon always pauses before he speaks......awkward moment.

"Sure, good idea." With the look of total understanding, he offered me a hug, then put his right hand on my right shoulder while he motioned Zac with his left, and they were on their way. I wrote:

> *Gratitude now. Deep gratitude today:*
> *for my heart which dares to speak to me;*
> *for a newfound willingness to listen;*
> *for the freedom of schedule clearing;*
> *for a young boy becoming man;*
> *for my needs and wants being heard as I try to hear the*
> *needs and wants of others;*
> *even for Dad's illness, in a strange way, for crystallizing*
> *the questions.*

I made my morning call, "Mom, I've decided not to go to New York today. We can hang out while Dad's having the cath. We can go to lunch, and then go see him later, if you want."

"Sue, you don't have to do this." Did I hear relief in her voice? She would never let me know. I sensed her trying to be strong.

"I know I don't have to. I want to."

6

Mom and I visited today and asked Dad, "What's going on? And what will they do tomorrow?"

He slowly shook his head, with that not-thinking look he gets before a golf shot. "You know, in the middle of a professional tournament, broadcasters ask the pros, 'What will you do tomorrow?' They always answer the same thing. They say, 'I'm going to do the same thing I did today. I'm going to go out there and be patient and let it happen.' So here I am. I am being patient and letting things happen. That's all I can do. We'll see soon enough."

SEVEN

REFRAMING

And I must admit that if I had to choose between a player with an excellent technique, but only a fair attitude, and another with a fair technique but a superior mental approach, I would take the latter every time.

Paul Runyan,
Book for Senior Golfers

Wednesday, June 23, 1999

A decision: By-pass surgery as soon as possible. Hopefully tomorrow. A week ago today, Zac, Mom, and I heard Dad's intuition, "I am a little concerned about my cardiac status." Now we realized the accuracy of his perception. The left ventricle was non-functioning from lack of blood flow. There was major occlusion in all the coronary arteries. Two of them were one hundred percent blocked, two others ninety-five percent blocked, and several smaller ones seventy-five percent blocked. As his heart muscle adapted to the lack of blood flow, it became enlarged. Dad's mitral valve was damaged as a result. Perhaps the surgeons would replace this vital tissue with a pig's valve, which would necessitate anti-rejection medications. As a minimum, the valve would be repaired, which would increase the length of "being under." Surgery was scheduled from eight in the morning until one in the afternoon, "if all goes well." Any complications, which were possible in a man of seventy-six with such a compromised heart, would extend surgical time and the danger. Dad would be on the heart and lung machine for several hours, at the very least, perhaps half a day. He would leave the operating room on a respirator, with several intravenous needles in his arms, legs, neck, and maybe belly, their long, connecting plastic tubes leading to bags full of various fluids. Machinery and technology would surround him, as he would be hooked to monitors all around his bed. After surgery, he'd be wheeled to the Special Care Unit (SCU), where he'd rest until stable enough for the next step. The medical team told us to prepare ourselves. Dad was not a good surgical risk. Yet surgery was the only real choice.

"Prepare yourselves," the words rang in our beings. I wondered what that meant, exactly. Prepare yourselves.

Thus ended a long week. It was only the beginning. Just when we were sure we could manage no more, we were being asked to delve deeper. I assumed preparing ourselves meant to dig down, go inside and pull out every ounce of strength available to us. Tools, skills, techniques, prayers, what did I have to help me through? No answers. After hearing the decision for surgery, I went to see Dad.

His room was filled with flowers; fresh daisies, withered daffodils, green plants with tiny get well cards stuck in the soil, hand-painted pictures in primary colors on the wall from Nicola and Antonio, his two toddler-ish great-grandchildren. In addition there was extra white bedding folded in a pile at the edge of the windowsill, topped with one folded blue and green floral Johnny. On the movable cart now positioned above his legs sat a brown plastic water pitcher sweating from the newly added ice cubes. Next to it in a foggy-colored cup remained watered-down ginger ale, now even paler yellow, with a bent plastic straw. "This room is a mess," my mother would later say, puttering about, fixing things up.

⑥

"Open heart surgery? This is great news." Dad was jubilant. "These are the best doctors in the country. Did you know that Maine Medical Center was just chosen #3 in the top hundred cardiac hospitals in the United States? I'm thrilled they can do something about my condition. They told me I'm a good surgical risk because I don't smoke, I'm not overweight, I've been active all my life, I'm not a drinker, and I don't have diabetes. Aside from this heart, I'm in great shape, they tell me. This is a remarkable team."

⑥

Just like golf. "You hit a shot and you think it's garbage. It's in the rough, or maybe it's even a lost ball and you need to take a penalty stroke. That may turn out to be the best thing that happens to you on the course that day. Maybe a shot like that can slow your game down, help you focus more. It can certainly help get rid of any cockiness, and get you humble again. Golf is a game of humility. You can have a day of hitting one great shot after another, but then when you hit a bad one—and you will—it can really throw you off. You gotta stay humble out there, or your mental approach can kill you. So a bad shot just might turn out to be a good thing."

He told *Maine Golf Magazine*, "I don't play that many tournaments any more; and what you lose is getting angry at yourself, which you have to do. You start reapportioning your time differently as you get older; a lot of things that were important to me in the past are very insignificant now…a missed three-foot putt doesn't bother me anymore."

🍃

Dad: a master at looking at things in many different ways. At Mt. Cranmore in New Hampshire, when Mom and Dad were teaching all seven us the tricks of down hilling, we'd ski and trip, run the boards a bit then catch a tip. Our tempers flew. Too overwhelmed to stand upright again, bundled as we were in thick scarves and heavy mittens, red leather Arlberg straps wrapped several times around our floppy lace-up ski boots, we cried. Hiding my red face in my ski gloves, I felt shame. Mark threw poles and swore. Ann pleaded to quit. Scurrying from the other side of the slope, skating with his poles, drawing herringbones with his skis, Dad responded with a bounce in his step and a smile on his ruddy face. "Wow! That was the best tumble I've seen all day. I wonder if you could do that again, just like that. I bet you can't crash that well a second time. Come on, show me another great fall."

Laughing now, we'd get up, brush ourselves off, and take to the slopes again. Dad fascinated us with this possibility; whether we saw these accidents as problems or as opportunities to have fun was not related to the fall; it depended on our attitude. Our happiness depended, we were learning from Dad, on how we framed things in our minds.

🍃

Several years after he retired from his oral surgical practice, Dad learned the art of framing. He fitted colorful borders and wooden casings on pictures that had never been finished before, and reframed old photos. In a small, well-lit passageway, between the lower level den and his woodworking shop in his basement, was Dad 's "frame shop." It began in the early

1980s when he bought a picture for $35.00 and decided to have it professionally matted.

"Dr. Lebel, the estimate for a single mat will be $12.50. A double mat will be another $12.50." Mom and Dad chose a frame, and left. The total bill for materials and labor for this $35.00 picture was over $60.00. Dad had been a surgeon, and wood-working had been a hobby for almost forty years. He had used tiny scalpels in surgery, and fine cutting edges to fit Formica. Self-assured, he committed to a new mission, "I can learn to mat and frame pictures."

His basement frame shop had a wall full of mat cutters, hanging from corkboard above a carpeted surface he used for fitting. Underneath were drawers full of knives, and scraps of oak and cherry from carpentry projects. There were various sizes and colors of matting material, some salvaged from past projects, some bought in bulk. Not only could he now fix up any inexpensive print he happened to purchase; he had also become a master at reframing.

It became a family joke. On a visit to their Florida winter home, I brought, as a house gift, a pair of line-drawn watercolor cartoons. Little likenesses of golfers. Very tiny. Very sweet. When my parents unwrapped the gift box, Mom laughed, "Oh, no, not more pictures, your father has been doing so much reframing that we have no room left on our walls."

"Of course, she's exaggerating," I thought.

But no. As he had practiced on the ski slopes and golf links, Dad had developed the habit of making things look better. Everywhere throughout their home, the reframed products of Dad's new craft decorated the walls. Indeed, there was not even an inch for these two tiny prints.

"Isn't this an improvement?" He proudly displayed an old ready-to-be-trashed photo, which was newly outlined by at least

one fresh mat. He also taught himself the skill of double matting, which presents any material in a whole new light.

All seven of us began sending him shots of our children,
"Dad, can you reframe THIS?"

Although his art projects piled up, the answer was always,
"Yes, sure, it'll look a lot better with a new frame."

(6)

Situational psychological reframing does not involve the materials, the hardware or the space that Dad's basement shop required. Putting events in perspective does require the same
precision, accuracy, steadiness, and clear thinking to create more
expansive frames of reference, to perceive our lives more accurately. I visited Dad on what we all expected to be his last day
before open-heart surgery. I brought him a special smooth, flat
stone to hold in his hands, a piece of the Earth, something solid.
As surgeon, woodworker, reframer, and golfer, his tactile sense was
well-developed. I imagined using his hands might be soothing. This
pale green, striated stone had a little hollow indentation which
provided a perfect groove for the thumb to slide back and forth.
With wide eyes, and "we'll take care of you, Mom, don't worry"
attitudes, Alisa and Zac had proudly handed me this very stone
the day before I faced major surgery thirteen years earlier. My children were ages three and five then, and they wanted me to know
this tiny rock would help me think of them while I was sick. "Mom,
you're not going into that operation without us," they hugged me
good-bye. "Hold onto this and we'll be with you." They coached
me to stroke it all day. "It's a lucky stone," were their last words to
me before they left the hospital.

(6)

I remembered the family story of Dad wearing his "lucky
socks," regardless of how gritty, sweaty and dusty they became,
from the beginning of a golf tournament until the last putt was

sunk. He would not let his mother wash or change his filthy, often argyle, socks until the end of the event, no matter how long it lasted. Suspecting that Dad was somewhat superstitious, I figured he would appreciate a lucky stone.

⑥

Sitting in my cherry nightstand drawer for thirteen years, this rubbing piece now had a new usefulness; to remind Dad that he was not going into surgery alone. I presented the green charm, and recounted the story my children had told me.

Instantly, he took to the good luck stone. "It's so easy to rub, and it feels great. I hope I don't break it."

"Oh, no you won't, Dad. It's rock solid. It won't break. Why don't you just hold it in your hand for a while, if it feels good to you? You look tired now. Mom and I can go to lunch, and you can nap. We'll see you in about an hour."

"Okay." He dozed off, right hand massaging the green amulet.

When Mom and I returned from our half-eaten lunch, the hospital room bustled. Ann stood at the foot of the bed with two eleven-year-old cousins; Sarah, her own daughter, and Jenny, Vicki's daughter. The young girls shied away from their Pepere, now ashen, thin, and slumped. Ann, dressed in business attire, with makeup for work, looked pretty there at the end of the bed, no doubt an outer persona for the girls, for Dad, for her job. Her dark hair was shiny, picking up light from the sunny window, but her hesitancy revealed that she, too, felt the same way we did. Ann was clearly pulled between comforting the girls and moving toward Dad.

Dad's younger sister, Anita, sat on the window side of the bed in a big green plastic chair. Twelve years his junior, she visited daily, some days offering gifts of chocolate or perhaps a card. Each day, she delivered news of their hometown, Lewiston.

As if to calm her own nervousness about her big brother's condition, she chewed gum and detailed the news of this cousin, that golf tournament. I joined her, jumping onto the cluttered windowsill. Mom squeezed in on the other side of the bed, maneuvering around the lunch tray and the drawn curtain. Dad smiled, "I've been rubbing this stone since you left."

"SNAP!" Like any golfer whose ball has just whacked a tree on an approach shot, Dad's eyes darted open, his forehead lines deepened, his face flashed crimson, and he bolted upright in bed. "Oh, my God, I broke the worry stone."

Sarah and Jenny froze. Ann and Mom whipped toward to Anita, now gasping, face covered in her hands. Anita, her perfectly bobbed salt and pepper hair now flinging around her small face, fired her piercing eyes at mine, as if to say, "Do something, Susan. Now!"

My mind flashed, "Time for a reframe."

"Oh, Dad, this is PERFECT! No, no, it's not a worry stone. It's a lucky stone. Lucky stones are meant to be passed on and on, and to be massaged until they split. They're supposed to break. That's a very good sign. It means you've got all the luck out of that stone. I have more at home, that's what they're for. In fact I have another one right here in my purse." I was indeed carrying a favorite shell, with the same type of thumb indentation, handy for rubbing in stuck traffic or in line at the bank. "Here, take this one. It's good luck to end one and…it's good luck to start one."

Later, Anita exclaimed, "Wow, that was good. How did you come up with that so fast?"

Easy. I learned it from Dad on the ski slopes.

6

Mike returned from Maui, jet-lagged, entered his house, and his children reported about Dad. Dropping his luggage, Mike dashed to the hospital to be with Dad before the next day's surgery. Since Dad had retired thirteen years ago, Mom and Dad had depended on Mike for estate planning. Among talk of Hawaii and vacationing, Mike assured Dad that his finances were fine, that there was no business left unfinished, and that Dad didn't have to worry about any of it.

Mike is bald like Dad, in constant motion like both Mom and Dad, built physically more like Dad, short, compact. His frame and personality are wiry; he talks fast, walks faster, thinks faster still, and is full of jokes. His energy moves outward, hands extended to greet and welcome whoever shows up. Charm oozing, Mike invites smiles. He delivered his business message to Dad quickly, concisely, in order to get to the important stuff— Hawaiian golf.

Dad was comforted by Mike's optimism, and thankful to hear the good financial news. He added, "Mike, I'm not going anywhere. I'm just really tired from all this waiting around and I'm ready to get going. I'm glad they can fit me in so soon, because the anticipation is beginning to get to me. I'm not really scared. I just want to get this over with and behind me, and the sooner the better. I'm delighted it's tomorrow."

Mike sensed the expectancy. At the very moment Dad finished confiding in Mike about his pleasure to be on the schedule first Thursday morning, Dad's cardiac surgeon entered the room. Handsome, his confident presentation belied his teenage appearance. "Dr. Lebel, I'm sorry to have to tell you that there have been some emergencies on this floor. We've had to postpone your surgery. Now we hope it can be Friday, but if not, it'll be Monday for sure."

Dad pursed his lips, and ran his right hand across the top of his freckled head. He hesitated, inhaled. A loud silence filled the room. Within seconds, however, he breathed out, "Okay."

There was another pause. The white-coated surgeon leaned forward and opened his mouth to speak. As steady as in his consistent pre-shot routine, Dad said, "Well, it's okay. I'm kind of disappointed that I won't be getting this over with tomorrow, but if putting me off can help someone else, then that's a good thing. I'm happy about that."

@

Dad placed his mind carefully in golf. "You don't get up to the tee and think, 'I hope I don't hit the water. Oh, no! I know I'm going to go straight to the water. Oh, please don't let this land in the water.' Instead you step up to the ball every time, the same way each time, with an 'I can do this' confident attitude. You expect the shot to go well. You address the ball. You plant your feet, square your hips and shoulders. You check your grip. You feel the club in your hand, see how it moves. You can only hit this one shot you're hitting, so you have to leave the bad news of the last shot behind. Then you put your attention on where you want the ball to go and you rotate your body around that ball. Same thing every time. You take a solid hit through the golf ball. Focus on the fundamentals. Don't focus on the hazards. Keep your mind positive. Swing and let it go. Let it happen."

@

He turned the disappointing postponement into an optimistic viewpoint: his delay would help others. In golf, when fans marveled at how long Dad hit his drive, he always offered the same reframe, "It's not how far; it's how many. Golf is not as simple as good tee shots. The game is complex, and there are many circumstances, tee-to-green, that need to come together for consistent shot making, and eventual success."

With Dad's reframing, now I understood: it was not how long we waited for his surgery; it was how all the circumstances would come together for an eventual success. I put my attention on how I wanted it to go, and let it happen.

As he has done all his life, Dad reframed. As if he weren't the "sick one," but rather in his familiar place on the top of the leader board, he taught the rest of us the way. Same thing every time.

EIGHT

TRUSTING

To have courage for whatever comes in life—everything lies in that.
St. Theresa of Avila

Thursday, June 24, 1999

My stomach turned. I sat for meals; it turned more. There were lumps in my throat. I didn't sleep. Restless dreams were my bed companions. Dad also reported that, even with sleeping medication, he tossed and turned from midnight on. A big question pervaded my being, "How will I say good-bye to Dad?"

Surgery had been scheduled. Friday at 6 a.m., the operating room staff would begin preparation: shaving Dad's gray-haired chest, cleaning all the hair from his once-muscled legs and arms. This day the surgeon and the anesthesiologist would read him everything that could possibly go wrong and remind him of the seriousness of his condition. We would be told the next day that the surgical team had debated whether to perform this surgery at all; that his heart was so diseased, and the muscle so weak that many surgeons wouldn't have touched him. Those were their exact words. "Wouldn't have touched him." These remarks were not uttered to us before the surgery, but we knew. We knew from this week of careful testing. We knew from the several terrifying diagnoses that resulted. We knew from his age and his family history. Yes, he had been stable for five days. Yes, other than his heart, he was a strong man. One of his cardiologists would later reveal, "This man has strong protoplasm, and that's important in this business."

I wondered if his protoplasm would outweigh the surgical risks.

Surgery would begin at 8 a.m. My thoughts wavered from one extreme to another.

"This is my last day with my Dad. Forever."

That conviction triggered the internal haunting and questioning. "How do I say good-bye for the last time ever?" And then my mind flipped to "Oh, well, just a little common bypass surgery. It happens in hospitals all over the country every day. There are five or six performed daily in this hospital alone. Maine Medical Center is one of the best hospitals for cardiac care. There's a saying around here, 'if you're going to have heart troubles, this is the place to be.' Ho, hum, just a little routine open heart surgery."

✿

I begin every morning with a period of meditation; this day was no exception. To end my quiet time, I repeat several lines, a practice from ancient Buddhism. These wishes invoke kindness toward myself and send hope and friendliness to others. Daily I offer this lovingkindness; being friendly seems crucial for all of us. Anytime. This day this practice was imperative. Some days, this ritual becomes rote, mechanical, automatic, and repetitive. This particular morning the phrases had new strength. Today their meaning permeated as I recited them:

May I be at peace.
May I have physical happiness.
May I have mental happiness.
May I have ease of well-being.

I repeated them for Mom, and for the family:

May we be at peace.
May we have physical happiness.
May we have mental happiness.
May we have ease of well-being.
May I be happy......May Mark be happy....may Ann be happy....may Mike be happy....may Vicki be happy....may Dave be happy....may Paul be happy....may Mom be happy....

And I sent well-wishes to Dad and his protoplasm:

May Raymond be at peace.
May Ray have physical happiness.
May Dad have mental happiness.
May he have ease of well-being.

I hoped for courage, but a gray cloud loomed. Do some people, I wondered, maintain steady optimism and consistency throughout? I doubted it. I suspected everyone had both hints of faith then stretches of no faith, and that they appeared and disappeared moment-to-moment. In this family, we had all had flashes of bright sunny outlook, and then the storms of fear. The human mind does funny things at times like this.

I asked Mike, "What's going on for you?"

Since Mike was a bouncy, wiry, energetic toddler, he has always moved with wit and quickness and jocularity. He has never been a sit-down-and-talk-about-it kind of guy. Today he quipped, "I don't like to think about it."

We were, perhaps afraid to think, because the mind might wander to the places of the faithless. Mike had visited Mom and Dad regularly, had often taken Dad boating. When Dad retired, Mike began the business preparing himself for Dad's death, he told me one day at lunch. It is the nature of his work, Mike claims, to "amortize feelings over time." But right now he didn't like to think about it.

I wondered about Vicki, too. Vic is golf-competitive like Dad, physically strong, focused; a woman of many talents. Still in California, she phoned often. Feeling mostly at ease, Vicki's only source of information was the upbeat news she'd hear from Dad, with his attitude of gratitude, his reframing. Vic, too, suffered moments of diminishing faith. "Thinking we'd played our final rounds of golf together was the worst," she confided when she talked to me on her return.

Vic had caddied for Dad in tournaments; Dad had caddied for her in the finals of the Portland County Club Championship. They shared golf videos, golf stories, golf books, and many Father-Daughter tournaments. Vic was perhaps thinking the worst as she remembered the best.

Mom worried, "What if he never comes back and sits in this living room again?"

Even as she asked, I could visualize them both in that space, filled with various silver Revere bowls, trophies, walls covered with pictures of Dad and his golf buddies. Golf videos labeled, *Better Golf*, and stacks of *Golf Digest* and the *New England Journal of Golf* hide beneath the television cabinet, behind the closed doors of the wooden entertainment center.

Normally, after dinner, Mom and Dad rested—he in his creamy gray leather recliner, her in her green leather arm chair—

watching the local half hour of news, then Dan Rather or Tom Brokaw, then the national talk shows. Every evening for years now, they had relaxed together; shared ice cream together right before bed. She closed the drapes at the same time every night; he was often asleep in his corner. Usually they didn't talk much after these fifty-plus years of marriage. Some nights they argued about the controversial guests on the *O'Reilly Factor*. Between ten and eleven o'clock, she hustled out to the driveway for her final cigarette of the day, returning afterwards to the gray and pink living room to announce, "Come on, Ray, it's time for bed." After this many years, relationship had grown into love and ritual and habit. Their history cut a deep trough, well-worn so that their separate streams had joined. How could Mom's mind possibly wrap itself around the idea of the loss of what was now part of her? With Dad gone from that chair, not sitting in that living room ever again, she would be as an amputee.

⑥

This family was caught in hesitancy, wanting to believe, yet holding our breath. *May we be at peace. May we have physical happiness. May we have mental happiness. May we have ease of well-being.*

My mind scanned for people who might embody being at peace, who were physically healthy, mentally healthy, and at ease in the world.

My daughter.

Although Alisa's hair is dark, unlike Dad's red, she inherited her grandfather's build; not too tall, athletic, freckled. She shares his temperament; optimistic in the face of hardship, resilient under most circumstances, with a general lifeway of meeting challenges head on. Just as Dad announced with total conviction, "I never enter a golf tournament I don't expect to win," so Alisa had traveled to developing countries with the total conviction that all would work out for the best. Just as Dad quieted himself, dug deep inside to pull out the golf game he needed in any moment, so Alisa meets the outside world, excavating deep inside herself for the resources to create a "win."

They both shoot high. I remember when I was a little girl, coming home one day from school to find Dad replacing the old harvest gold colored kitchen counter tops with new cream-colored Formica. Not aware that he knew anything about such work, I asked, "Dad, how did you learn to do that?" He answered, so matter-of-factly, "I got an estimate of what would cost to have this replaced, and when I got the quote, it was outrageous, so I said to myself, 'I can learn this.'" He did.

In like manner, Alisa decided in high school at North Yarmouth Academy to try out for the Varsity Girls' Hockey team. She had never skated. Dad asked her, "Alisa, how can you play hockey at NYA if you don't know how to skate?"

With *his* characteristic poise, she answered, "Pepere, I can learn."

She did.

He had recounted this tale again and again. Each time he leaned back in his chair, lifted his feet off the ground, opened his mouth wide, lunged out his tongue and raised his eyebrows. Her moxie delighted and surprised Dad. "I get such a kick out of that story," he beamed and chuckled every time in the re-telling.

⑥

I do not understand Dad's not understanding Alisa. Dad was not a man filled with self-doubt. On the golf course he taught, "The worst thing you can do is to doubt yourself, to doubt how you read the ball. You have to decide what you're going to do with your shot—what club, where to hit it, how far, how high. You have to know where you want to go. Then you visualize it, and commit to your choice. Once you commit to your shot, you can't be saying 'Gee, maybe I should hit it a little more left,' or 'maybe I should use a seven iron instead of this eight.' Once you make your decision, there is no more thinking, no more questioning. The mind is off. You put your hands on the grip and address the ball. You step up and strike the ball the way you planned."

The dictionary defines faith as "confidence or trust; belief which is not based on proof." Golfers with confidence believe they can make it around the course with the fourteen allowed clubs; people who trust have minds that more easily settle down, and stop questioning. I needed more grounding than I had in my bag, so I called Alisa.

Some people nicknamed Dad "Golden Boy," for everything he touched created success—his career, his horn playing, his family, his carpentry, his golf. I had given birth to his grand-daughter, a veritable "Golden Girl." Alisa, like Dad, never entered a game she did not expect to win. As her mother, I'd love to take credit for her sparkling essence; truth is, she arrived in the world full of it. Her second grade teacher, Lisa, declared, "A day without Alisa in school is like a day without sunshine."

This summer she lived and worked in Bar Harbor, a small Maine coastal town, enjoying her short two months between NYA graduation and her first year at Middlebury College. I was happy for her and yet I missed her.

I phoned her to hear her energetic voice, "Hi, Mom," were her usual first words. Before she answered, I anticipated the familiar tone and that smile on her face on the other end of the line. We were close as mother and daughter and I wanted her near me now, if only by voice. I told myself that I was calling her to relate that surgery was scheduled for the next day. I called her, in fact, to connect, to think aloud. I called her because I knew she'd cheer me up. I called my daughter because, even though I had none, I wished for courage.

"Hi, Mommy!" She overflowed with news of her summer.

We chatted briefly. Words sticking in my throat, I began to tell her about Pepere, and what tomorrow would bring. She hesitated. Her voice lowered. "Well, Mom, do people die when they have this surgery?"

The question hit like a swift punch, the impact knocking me back.

"Well, sure they do. Just not often…hardly ever. I know this medical team wouldn't do the surgery if they thought that would happen. Alisa, you wouldn't believe how good these doctors are. Pepere keeps saying, 'They are remarkable.' And the surgeons are very skilled. They're performing this surgery so Pepere will feel better than ever soon."

"So, most people survive this, huh?"

She confronted the tough uncertainties I dared not speak.

"Oh, sure. In fact, we heard yesterday that statistics are heavily in his favor for a great result at the Maine Medical Center."

She stepped into her usual positive stance. "Well, then, Mom, this is a good thing. His heart will be stronger, and he'll have more energy."

"Oh, yea, it's definitely a good thing. He's going to be fine."

⑥

As I heard my words of encouragement for Alisa, I felt my terror softening. Worry abated about how to speak to Dad. Perhaps preparation for a final "good-bye" could be replaced by "see ya' later."

We grow in connection with other people, and reaching out sends hope, simultaneously, to both ourselves and to others. I

told Alisa what I needed to hear. I said to her what I most wanted
to believe. I had abandoned hope, but speaking with my daughter restored faith. Optimism is infectious. I began to trust.

NINE

RELATING

It is highly moral people, unaware of their other side, who develop peculiar irritability...which make them insupportable to the relatives.

Carl Jung

Friday, June 25, 1999

Day of Surgery, the ninth day of our hospital vigil. On other scorching Maine summer Friday mornings, Dad played golf with his "Friday group." Between 11:00 and 1:00 they gathered at the Portland Country Club, sometimes eighty players for their informal weekly tournament. Often, money was bet for closest to the pin, or most birdies, or skins. Each player threw in $15.00 to enter, then the fun began. For the past fifteen years, Friday's action, once called "The Swindle," kept Dad and his buddies Mike, Al, Frank, Dick, and Tommy, laughing, teasing—all to walk away, at most, with an extra ten or twenty dollars in cash prizes.

"Ray's taken more money out of there than anybody over

the years," chided longtime, friendly competitor Mike. "But it's not for the money. We're all great friends. It's an honor to play with Ray. He's the classiest guy. You never hear him get mad. He never uses vulgarity or curses. He's taught all of us a lot about being a gentleman. If he has a bad hole or a big score, you'd never know it. He just keeps on playing and most of the time ends up with the best score anyway at the end of the day."

When the play ended, the golfers gathered in the locker room for more kidding, drinks, and a little food. There was one other very short break, a hurried rest; after playing the front nine, and before playing the back nine. At the halfway point of their round, the men stopped briefly to grab a hot dog and scramble to the tenth tee. Outside the Grill Room were other foursomes, and there was quick friendly banter. "Did you see how far back the tee was on three?" or "The greens are in great shape today, aren't they?" or maybe, "How're ya' hittin' em?" And, perhaps, "the play is so slow."

Between the front nine and the back nine, there was barely enough time for a bathroom break, to wipe the accumulated sweat from the morning's heat, to connect with others playing the same course, or to refresh before meeting the remaining challenge. Golfers keep the play moving and get back on the course in order not to lose their spot.

🌀

Today, the ninth day, we would bear a seemingly unbearable challenge, surgery. We shared the same rushing in our cells that the Friday group experienced. Finishing the ninth hole, starved for a leisurely lunch, their cleated feet dashed off to the tenth tee. We too could benefit from stopping, taking a breath, resting before what lie ahead, yet time did not halt for us any more than for the steady line of weary, hungry golfers. It would be as emotionally hot inside this air-conditioned hospital, as the sun would be on the steamy links. Driving to MMC, we noted the perfect warm summer greens outside, which only heightened the contrast with hospital sterile whites and its silver needles.

⑥

Surgery would begin at 8 a.m. Dad's surgeon, Dr. Weldner, informed us that he was first on the schedule because the he liked to "get the tough ones over with early." As family, we had received our instructions. We were to be in the Special Care Unit (SCU) waiting area. The doctor wouldn't see us until it was over, but we would get details from staff midway through the procedure. Our job was to wait.

We arrived at the hospital at 9:30. Maybe 9:30 would be about the middle, we figured. Dad was wide open on a surgical table. A knife culled his legs for veins. Kept alive on a heart and lung machine, he would receive units of whole blood and platelets. The experts admittedly could not predict in advance whether they would find three or more arteries that needed replacing. Several times, we were warned of the possible necessity of adding another hour and a half for a mitral valve replacement.

Like getting familiar with the layout of the course, we paced the SCU waiting room. It was decorated with soft chairs, lovely pastel watercolors hanging on the cream-colored walls. For our convenience, a tan wall phone was tucked in a visible corner. The rich aroma of freshly brewed coffee wafted through the room, as coffee and tea pots sat on a metal server. Next to them, icy juices in silver pitchers produced beads of cold water sweating down the sides. Volunteers replenished bakery-made blueberry muffins, too big for one person to eat.

We were comfortable and we were uncomfortable simultaneously. Our chests were heavy, throats tight, guts in knots.

Families gathered, each in their own area, huddled together, whispering. Still, we heard. Even murmured conversations rang out in this intense setting. Each cluster had a loved one in grave danger, as SCU offered the most critical care that medicine provides. Patients in SCU were the most life-threatened, the closest to death. Families waiting for news were understandably edgy.

Eyes darting around the tense room, I watched the families. Behavior varied widely. In one group, a full-bellied, maybe eighty-year-old male wearing scuffed black orthopedic shoes, hobbled, bent over a cane, cigarettes rolled into his white t-shirt sleeve. His wife jumped up and down around him, perhaps protecting him, and rushed to receive any information. She then quietly filtered it through people I assumed to be sons and daughters. Finally they spoke to the frail man.

In another more boisterous family, a teenage son sobbed openly, while the twenty-something daughter skulked around the room and yelled at her tearful mother, "I can't be here this summer to help you. How many times do I have to tell you? I 'm moving to the lake!"

A woman who could have been this young woman's grandmother hopped up every time the phone rang. In a shaky voice, she announced the name of the person being called. "Is anyone from the Smith family here?" She then paced the long well-lit hallway outside the SCU waiting area until the phone conversation ended, at which time she scurried to make a call.

Another group of three people fidgeted in the corner. The only male, with skinny tattooed arms, sat with an oxygen tank next to him, hooked to a tiny plastic tube leading to his nostrils. One of the permed-haired women glanced furtively each time a new person entered the room. Disgusted, another prattled all morning, "You know these doctors don't know what they are doing. I know someone who sued a surgeon because he mutilated his leg."

Two seventy-ish women froze in stone silence across from one another in the back corner. They made no eye contact. I sensed they were quarreling cousins, or spatting siblings who had refused to speak for years. A mutual relative was on a nearby operating table, so here they were together.

Just down the hallway from this large reception area filled with family scenarios was a smaller room, designated for conferences with the doctors. The cozy space was designed like a den with homey furniture, oriental carpets, colorful art work with gold-gilded frames, and table lamps providing soft, yellow lighting. Every now and then during the morning, someone official dressed in surgical blues, little round caps on their heads and cotton slippers on their feet, appeared, asking, "Could the Jones family come to the special meeting room, please?"

Mom commented, "A consultation away from this big group probably means upsetting news. No doubt, the nurses don't want to deliver bad news in this big, public waiting area in front of all the other families."

We dreaded being called to that attractive den. We hoped it would be possible to receive our reports right here.

Camaraderie developed among the small diverse crowds in this room we inhabited this morning. Curious, we inquired, "What are you here for?"

In this community, as each family's drama played out, we cared. One young woman waited to hear about her mother, who had lapsed into a coma. No one yet knew why. Two other families also had loved ones in open heart surgery. Another had suffered a near-fatal car accident. The phone rang, the room hushed, and we strained to hear the tone and see the expression on faces as relatives received calls. We were all in this together.

We had gathered—Mom, Dave, Anita, and I at first. Mark and Ann would join us at lunch. Paul was to call us, and we would call him at work as the day progressed. Vicki was in California, staying in touch by phone. Mike was at work, we'd been told. Anita had brought the sweater and the pattern she created. Her nervous fingers knitted and purled all morning. Needles clicked. Mom and I carried books, although our level of unease left them unread. Dave talked nonstop. We were exhausted. Yet we were only beginning our vigil on this, the steepest and fastest section of the roller coaster. This upside-down-disoriented-scream-producing ride was happening on the steamiest day of the year—both literally and figuratively. Outside it was ninety-five degrees, and humid. In SCU Waiting Area #1, we were even hotter under the collar. With the highest level of anticipation yet, we relieved the pressure our emotions generated. Mom left occasionally for a cigarette. I kept leaping up to make calls. Anita finished more rows, and chomped gum. Dave entertained with loud "Dirty Ernie" jokes, and our hilarity may have been inappropriately uproarious.

At about 10:30, a nurse from the surgical team, with a little folded notepaper in her hand, found us. Anita's hands and all the nervous comedy halted. Directly from the operating room, our messenger sat down in this living room squarely across from our pained faces, with a smile on hers. We made the assumption, therefore, that what she had to say would be okay to hear in this space. "So far, everything's going well. He went on the heart and lung machine well, and if there's going to be trouble, sometimes it starts right there. We've already fixed four arteries and it looks like we'll have to do more. The valve can probably be repaired rather than replaced, but we don't know for sure yet. He's doing fine. I'll come back to talk with you near the end. Then when it's all over, the doctor will speak with you."

Tears swamped our eyes. Faces flushed. We breathed again. Our own hearts quickened; the adrenaline of relief pulsed through us. We clutched each others hands with a collective "augh." I lunged to the phone to call the others. When I returned to the seats, we waited for relatives to gather, and our own saga began. Everybody in the room was spent, and each one of us manifested it differently:

This one was furious with that one for not being here, and the gossip flew. Another one of us blurted. "They should be here."

This was easy, to join the judging. What was difficult was feeling the fear of mortality and the anger at our human dilemma. We did what frazzled people often do; we projected it. We complained. "What's the matter with that one?"

"I can't believe they did that, can you?"

One person reprimanded the rest us, "Look, this is no time for a family feud."

Showing up for a few minutes at lunch, one sibling breezed in, told a few jokes, and breezed out. We criticized that one, too.

Another arrived at lunch with a headache and fear of oncoming panic.

Yet another one of us had brought old family albums, and wanted us to sit and page through them now. No one could be still long enough to look

Someone wanted to smooth everything over. We shouldn't make it bigger than it was.

Some of us were quiet, some vociferous.

None of this struck me as dysfunctional. Indeed, we were functioning well, whatever that meant. We were doing the best we could under the most pressing of circumstances. These were the dynamics of a family on watch. Perhaps we were releasing the tension we felt with the people we loved the most; this family was safe.

We came together, emotions raw and on the surface, fear running deep underneath. Dad was on a table right at that moment, chest broadly opened, wide plastic tube down his throat. Dad would not want the family heart struggling now. Dad was a "if you can't say anything nice, don't say anything at all" guy. He could be tough when he needed to be, in tournaments or when his sense of fairness was crossed, but he was the one who cried at tender poems and at family anniversaries when heartfelt Hallmark cards were read aloud. He would want our hearts to be open.

⑥

In college I asked Dad, "Dad, I'm going to a keg party and I don't drink. They want $5.00 from everyone to cover the cost of the keg, but don't you think I should just tell them I don't have to pay because I'm not going to have any beer?"

His answer was swift and sure. "Of course you'll contribute. You're going to the party, you'll be in the gathering and you have to pay. Sometimes being part of the group takes precedence over what you do for yourself."

⑥

This was one of those times. Being part of this family, supporting each other, rooting for Dad, took precedence over whether I thought this brother should have been here or this sister should have come earlier. Of course, we had to pay. We paid homage to this man, who taught us, even in his illness, how to be part of this group. So we made peace inside ourselves, some with prayer, some with silence, and some with individual self-talk. We didn't apologize to each other; we said very little; we knew why we were here, so we felt our feelings, and we did what Dad would want us to do. We came together and we waited.

⑥

Dad is a realist, practical. One year, his golf buddies noticed that, from October through December, he had used only three golf balls. He hit the same ball, day after day, as it turned from white to gray. One afternoon, he walked in on them in the clubhouse as they were emptying their pockets. He asked, "What are you doing?"

They turned to him. "Ray, we're taking up a collection."

"Taking up a collection?"

They ribbed him. "We're taking up a collection to buy you a new golf ball."

"They don't get it," he told me.

I didn't really get it either. "Dad, why do you play with the same ball?"

"Well, you know I brought three dozen balls to Florida that fall, but I wasn't hitting into the water, so I just kept using the same ball. I don't care if my ball is dirty. I don't get any extra length out of a new ball any more, the way I play now. I can see, if I were Tiger Woods, I'd have to change a ball every three holes, because they decompress. For me now, why do I need a new ball?"

(6

We held his values with us as we waited. There had been times when Dad was on the golf committee at various clubs, when it had been reported that a certain golfer was cheating, changing scores, not taking penalty shots, or moving the ball for a better lie. He never understood this. "How can you feel good about your game if you're not playing fair? How can you feel good about yourself as a person if you cheat? What good is winning that way? You have to sleep with yourself at night, you know." When he first heard the news about the dishonesty, he was not inclined to do anything about the person cheating, as he believed, "That person will defeat himself eventually."

But when, in his role, he was called to act, Dad worked with a committee, gathered data, confirmed the facts, moved cautiously, often helping the one who cheated to save face. In the end, after all the consultation, he did what needed doing, and rendered a decision.

6

We knew we must play fair, act as a family, work with our little committee. We needed to gather the facts, and do what needed doing. No matter what might happen to him on the operating table, we would each have to sleep with ourselves tonight.

The ring of the tan wall phone interrupted our vignette. I snatched it. After listening, I asked the room, "Is there anyone from the Able family here...No?"

I returned to the caller, "No, not here."

The voice on the other end was demanding, so I offered, "Wait, I'll go to the other waiting area."

Not to be quieted, the caller screamed at me. I answered, "Yes, I know it's urgent. I'll run."

On my way out, I bumped against the shoulders of an oncoming woman in operating room garb who was rushing in. "Is there anyone in the room from the Nelson family? I want to see you down the hall in the little den."

Involved in my own drama, I nevertheless stopped, or was stopped by a force which clenched my body, hit hard by the vision of the Nelson family, hearing what they must hear in a little private, quiet space.

6

Perhaps half of our vigil was over. As if just finishing the front nine, Anita, Mom, Ann, Dave, and I took our hurried rest between the morning and the afternoon. We felt the press of time, and rushed for a bathroom break, to wipe the accumulated sweat from the morning's heat, to connect, and to refresh before meeting the challenge of the end of this day. We rode the elevator to the hospital gift shop and café. While trying to eat, we visualized Dad with tubes down his throat, not knowing whether his front teeth might have been knocked out, as the anesthesiologist suggested might happen during forceful intubation. We attempted brief friendly banter. We consoled one another. Dave picked up the tab. Internally, there was fear and relief of fear, hope and doubt, feelings of family connection and disconnection. Externally, we griped. "Look at these oozing globs of mayonnaise in the tuna salad. This can't be good for heart patients."

"This service is so slow."

And we grumbled that the table was filthy.

໑

Soon after lunch, a physicians' assistant informed us that the surgery was almost over, that seven arteries had been replaced, that the valve could be repaired. Dad was still doing fine. I knew Dad was being kept alive by machines right now. I knew he was closer to death in this instant than at any other in his life. Yet I was, in an unexplainable way, more relaxed than at any other time during this past week. Again, I marveled at the unpredictability of the human condition, and the paradox of the human mind.

Having survived our greatest stress, we were relieved, and exhausted. After six hours of surgery, the surgeon joined us in the main living room. "This man went through a lot today. We repaired seven arteries. This was very tricky, very risky surgery. Some surgeons wouldn't have touched him. Even the veins in his legs were too small, so we had to go deeper into the legs to find good ones. His arteries were horrible..... awful...terrible. Two of them were one hundred percent occluded, and two more ninety percent occluded. We repaired seven to give him plenty of blood flow. He's had lots of bleeding, and we've given him two units of blood. He's stable now, but…"

He broke eye contact, stared at the floor, shrugged his shoulders and lifted his upturned palms, "We'll just have to see."

Shocked, Anita and I shot terrified glances at each other, as if to ask, "What the hell does THAT mean? 'We'll just have to see'?"

The doctor added, "In about twenty minutes, you can see him in SCU if you want. Be prepared for all the tubes, the respirator, and the machines."

◈

The call came. "The Lebel family can go to SCU now to see Dr. Lebel." Mom pulled my hand. "I don't know if I should see him like that. What do you think?"

I didn't know. "Well, Mom, it depends. If you think you need to see him to prove to yourself that he's alive and made it through, then it's a good thing. If you're afraid that image of him on the respirator will haunt you all night, then don't. I'll go in and tell you how he looks, and you can come back later, or tomorrow."

"Susan, you do it," Mom was shaking, "then tell me if I should. I can't be first. You go."

I peeped into Dad's SCU cubicle. His body, which I knew to be all cut up, was covered in soft pastel blue cotton blankets. Only his head showed. Needles grew from his neck. A big plastic tube from the respirator draped from his wide open mouth. Taped to his forehead was a yellow plastic tube, surrounding him like a halo. Hanging from a large metal frame behind his head dangled plastic bags of various fluids. A full bag of red blood was suspended from its own frame on one side of the bed, drips of red falling through a transparent line into an intravenous needle leading to his arm. Another bag swung from the bottom of the bed: a catheter bag; empty. A TV-type monitor was mounted overhead, with seven print-outs displaying patterns. One read HR, heart rate. Another said BP, blood pressure. The others meant nothing to us. His color was sepia-toned, yet he was definitely recognizable as Dad. Terror transformed into relief, even as I reminded myself that these few postoperative hours were the most crucial. Will his lungs want to be weaned from the respirator? Will his newly-repaired heart kick in? I touched Mom, not sure if I needed her to hold my hand there next to Dad's resting body, or that I wanted to be there to hold hers. "It's okay, Mom. Come. It's okay."

We took turns. Dave, Anita, Ann, Mark, Mom, and me. Anita's face flashed bright red, and her emotions let loose. She stooped and sobbed in the corner. Ann began to feel faint, and fell back. Mom clutched one of my hands, while she held Dad's in her other. Explaining his mission to the nurse as he entered the room, Mark made a second round to answer a question which had just come to us, "Does Dad still have his front teeth?" Lifting Dad's parched lips, Mark assured his anesthetized body, "Hey, old man, you've got your centrals."

We exited: there was nothing more to do. Dad would maybe begin to wake up much later tonight, we were told. Walking down the long SCU hallway together, arms around shoulders, our little clan started to disperse. We mumbled, "Isn't it amazing what modern medicine can do?"

"Wow, they did SEVEN? I've never heard of seven before."

"He looks a lot better than I thought he would."

"Aren't we lucky to be here in Maine?"

"Look at this great artwork on the walls."

"I hate this heat."

"Wouldn't you think everyone would want to be here?"

©

On this, the day we most feared, we did what families do. We cried together. We laughed together. We ate together. We hugged one another and also pushed one another away. We leaned, one on the other, for support and wished there had been more. We enjoyed some parts of the day and hated others. We sat steadfast through pain and sorrow, wobbling with the yips. As individuals, we coped with our stress using the full spectrum of human strategies. Some of us enhanced the drama which already existed. Some tried to reduce it. Others denied it. We comforted and were mad at one another simultaneously. Truth is, we managed one breath at a time.

Dad would have entered the day as he enters every tournament, expecting to win. In golf, he would step up to the first tee, confident, address the ball, and hit the first shot. No matter where it went—to the green, in the soggy rough, on the wide-open fairway—he would walk right up to the next challenge and address that ball again, as if it were the first shot of the day, as if he had not hit ten thousand of these shots before. As his longtime friend Mike noted, "He is the classiest guy."

Dad had always predicted, "If you want to get to know someone, play golf with them. You can tell who's got a hot temper, who has a tough personality, who's a nice guy. Golf brings out the best and the worst in people."

So does sitting in a sweltering waiting room filled with frightened loved ones, imagining they may never touch their patient again. It brought out the best and the worst in us.

©

Dad was a champion, and champions conduct themselves in the same manner on the golf course and in a waiting room. When we wavered, when the family felt is if we were sinking to the bottom of a water hazard, he would have approached as a gentleman, reminded us to stay cool and offered his best shot, leading us out of troubled waters.

TEN

BREATHING

The world breaks everyone and afterward many are strong at the broken places.

Ernest Hemingway

Saturday, June 26, 1999 ∾ *First postsurgical day*

Once again, I was struck by the life-supports in Dad's dimly-lit SCU room. The endotracheal tube from the respirator had been removed from his throat, replaced by a plastic oxygen cannula in his nostrils. The central venous line was still in his neck, and peripheral lines led to his wrist and arms. A transfusion of packed red blood cells dripped to one arm from above his head. The monitor screen still printed out seven lines of information. Surrounded by paraphernalia, it would be easy to forget the person, Dad, in the mass of tubes, wires and bags. Eyes closed, Dad was curled in a fetal position, scarcely resembling the man who raised me. His head, face, and arms were clean-shaven. Almost baby-like, he nuzzled around his pillow.

☙

I believe, deep in my core, that the more there is steel, plastic, and machinery, the greater is the need for the human, for love, to equal to the technology. The less one looks like himself, then the more our soft side must balance the hardware. In the midst of hospital, critical care, sterile floors, and clinical terminology, we arrived one by one. Our responses shared a similar quality; a natural intuition to treat Dad, not only as shattered but whole. Our own breathing was not exactly slow and regular, but we refused to let his unshaven face, his wasted color, the smells in the room and the clicking of the machines break our spirits. This SCU cubicle was packed with metal, tubes, machines, and with hearts, some breaking, some strong, some connecting.

Paul stood at Dad's side as I entered. He was alone with Dad. His eyes darted around the room, scanning the flashing lights. Paul fidgeted, and then relaxed noticeably, shoulders softening, voice lowering, when other family members appeared. Unshaven, un-showered, scruffy hair on his neck, but otherwise bald, Paul told me Dave had just left. All week, Dave had visited Dad first in the morning—7:00 a.m. or so. By 7:30 every day this week, Dave was at Mom's. Dave said, "You only get so many chances to let people know you love them. Some day it'll be too late to give appreciation."

When he first saw Dad, Dave was shocked speechless. With the conviction that Dad could hear him no matter what, Dave offered, "Hey, Dad, you're doing great. Hang in there; we're all here for you. You know, you're a tough old bird, you've always been a tough son-of-a-gun."

Dad smiled and managed to retort, "I got that from you."

⑥

Paul not talking now, simply cradled Dad's hand. I joined Paul, who beamed, "He knew me. He was out like a light, but when I came in and took his hand, he squeezed it, and he said, 'Hi, Paul.' I knew he couldn't say much, but I asked him, 'Dad, how're ya' doin? Dad, how're ya' feelin'?' He even answered me with a few words. Then I told him we're all hoping he'll get out of here soon."

Paul shifted away from Dad's bed. I stepped in close. "Only a minute," the critical care nurse warned, "while he's in this Special Care Unit."

These precious instants would be all I'd be granted. I wanted them to matter. I wanted the reaching out of my heart to make a difference in the healing of Dad's. The nurses and doctors insisted he wouldn't remember this, that he required rest and sleep. We were not to bother him. I wondered how touch and conversation could bother. Surely, human relationship would be the only way to get through the hardware. As saline solutions, blood and oxygen coursed through Dad's body, what coursed through mine was a current of quick thoughts, rushes of feeling, and torrents of sensation. Witnessing Dad so worn, so yellow, head so swollen, body so shrunken, was excruciating.

@

In my feeble attempts to learn golf as a young girl, I made the same mistake over and over again. Dad would repeat, "You're forcing the ball. Don't try to help the process. The club face will lift the ball. Soft hands. Soft hands. Slow your swing down. Patience. Let the club do the work. "

But I could never do what seemed so counter-intuitive. Tightening my hold on the club, I wanted to lift the shaft a tad more, or pull it back just a smidgen. If only I could be a little craftier with my grip, perhaps I could coax the ball over that hill. With my cocked head, I even tried to steer the ball after impact.

@

And now my grip felt too loose; my hold was slipping. If only I could say just the right thing. If only I were craftier with words. I yearned to help this process of recovery and rush the game. It was counter-intuitive to let time and nature wedge Dad out of this sand trap.

With bone level fatigue I took deep breaths. In. Out. I let go and softened on the exhale to release clenched feelings, to quiet the busy mind, and to relax tension. Replacing Paul by Dad's side, I slipped his hand in mine, lightly, as he had taught me to initiate the grip of a club. I inhaled deep breaths before talking. I focused on his eyes. Then noticed that his arm was warm and hairless. Resting my hand under his, I was cautious not to rustle too much, so as not to upset all the needles. Not knowing if his heartbeat would respond to the comforting by slowing and stabilizing—it can happen with human touch— I was nevertheless convinced that this hand-holding was for both of us. I leaned down to whisper directly into in his ear.

"Hey, Dad, you did great."

"Oh, hi, Sue. Yea, that's what they say." He muttered.

"Dad, they did SEVEN."

"So they tell me."

"Dad, Jon says 'hi,' and the kids send their love."

"Okay."

Skill with his hands had provided not only his life's work, but also his life's favorite pastimes of golf, trumpet-playing and carpentry. I set a new, clean, white Titleist ball in his cupped fingers, and asked, "Dad, do you know what this is?"

"It feels like another good luck charm." He remembered.

"Right. Do you know what kind?"

The corners of his mouth turned up. "It feels like a golf ball."

I knew his fingertips would recognize those indentations. "Yup," I assured him.

When he was healthy, he took for granted the delicate sense perception of a skilled surgeon who knew one tissue from another by feel alone, and the touch of a craftsman's magical fingers, able to detect the slightest variation in wood. The day after seven hours of surgery, he sensed that he had a bright shiny white ball in his hand—but in this moment his faculties were, of course, far from accurate. "It doesn't feel round."

⑥

Just then I was relieved to see Vicki, who seemed relieved to see me. She chuckled at his being curled up on his side, tucked around the golf ball. I stepped out of the clinical space, and Vicki slid in.

"Hey, Dad, I'm back."

"Oh, Vic, how was your trip?"

Vic said, "California was great. I think I had an easier week than you did last week. Go back to sleep and get some rest now. I'll see you tomorrow."

"Okay. Thanks for coming in."

⑥

Ann and Mom arrived next. Ann tiptoed in, and looked at Dad, body covered in a blanket, only his head and neck visible. Ann, too, picked a focal point to steady her gaze—his arms and hands, tan from golf. To Ann's eyes, he didn't appear to be uncomfortable. Reassured, Ann laughed at his being nuzzled with the golf ball. She squeezed his hand, "I love you, Dad."

"I love you."

"Dad, you have a big yellow tube across your head. It looks like a halo."

"Do I have the same hairdo?"

⑥

Mom's visit was simple, also. Although she trembled at first before touching him in this arena of lines and tubes, she took his hand. Before she could speak, Dad glanced at her and said, "I love you."

She kissed his head, "I love you, too. It's good to see you awake."

Dad reported that his mouth was dry, his lips felt stuck together. Although he was quite nauseous, he asked for crushed ice. I am reminded of another story:

A young family goes out to dinner. Everyone orders, and then it is time for the five-year-old son. He turns to the waitress, "I'd like a hot dog."

The mother and father immediately interrupt and bark at the waitress, "He'll have roast beef and mashed potatoes with peas."

The waitress turns her attention to the young boy and asks, "What would you like on your hot dog?"

As the waitress walks off, the boy beams, "Hey, Mom and Dad, that person thinks I'm real."

⑥

So it was with Dad. Although he looked childlike, tucked around his favorite toy, we treated him as real. Mark ran to the hospital gift shop to buy lip balm. Mom walked to the nursing station to fetch crushed ice. I fed it to him through a straw. Vicki talked golf with him. Ann offered him the names of people who'd asked about him. Paul talked to him about his daughter, Chelsea. Dave sneaked in a couple of times a day.

⑥

After dinner, I felt compelled to return to Maine Medical Center. This heartfelt urge was illogical, as he was already in a heavy sleep. I mentioned my desire to my husband, who advised, "Well, go if you want, but know you're going for you and not for him, because he won't know you're there."

Common sense notwithstanding, I wanted to say goodnight

to my father, and in some way that I could not articulate, I was convinced it would matter to him.

I called Mom. She said, "Oh, Sue, you don't have to do that. He's down for the night already. We can go in together tomorrow."

But my decision had nothing to do with being practical. I had to see him. That's all. I pulled up to the huge hospital on the tall hill overlooking all of Portland just before the heavy automatic outside doors locked at 8:00 p.m. Dad's SCU nurse informed me that his blood pressure was unstable, that he'd been nauseous all day. Because of complications he would not be leaving SCU tomorrow. I nodded, in silent acknowledgment, and announced, "I'm just going in to say good night."

"There's no need to. He can't hear you."

I didn't believe that.

Breathing deeply now, rhythmically, I talked to him, not aloud, rather, in my head. Holding his hand in silence for about twenty minutes, I stood bedside and we communicated.

With eyes closed, I imagined my words traveling from my mind down the neck into my chest cavity, through my heart, then carried by the breath out my hand, into his hand, and ultimately into his real being:

"Dad, you had seven arteries done. Seven! That's one for each of us. Pretty amazing, huh? We were all pulling for you. I called Alisa in Northeast Harbor, and she said to say good luck And I called Zac at theater camp. Guess what? He got a part in *42nd Street*. You know? It's that play we went to see in Florida with him. It's a play within a play, remember? You loved the music. You kept tapping the beat through the whole show with your fingers, remember?… and you told us that Pepere taught you one of the songs on the trumpet years ago…Yes, I'm sure you told us that. …Well, Zac got the part of one of the play-wrights. .. Jon played golf today, but he didn't hit the ball well, so he really wants to talk to you about his game…and…and…."

ELEVEN

ACCEPTING

*.....If you are respectful by habit,
constantly honoring the worthy,
four things increase:
long life, beauty,
happiness, strength*

> Walt Whitman
> *Leaves of Grass,*
> *(VIII: "Thousands")*

Sunday, June 27, 1999 ~ *Second post-operative day*

Sleep eluded me. I tossed and turned with visions of Dad in that little room, hooked up to machinery, nauseous. I wondered whether he would experience more pain as the anesthesia wore off, whether waking up would be less comfortable than his drug-induced slumber. At 6:00 a.m., I drove to the Medical Center. Just as I had to say good night a few hours ago, now I wanted to say good morning.

As I approached the entrance to his room, I spotted a nurse next to him. Was her name badge hard to read, or was I not seeing straight? Squinting, I could barely make it out, with its tiny black letters under shiny clear plastic, backed in bright white. Was it Margaret, or Maggie, or, perhaps, Mary? I'll call her Mary. It appeared to me that Mary was rough with Dad, throwing his body from one side to the other, thrashing him around. She was neither gentle nor friendly. The reactive part of me would have shouted, "Hey, watch it there, Mary, what do you think you're doing? Be careful, he's just had open heart surgery, you know."

Of course, I knew she knew. It also occurred to me that she might be doing exactly what she was supposed to be doing. My perception was a bit skewed, perhaps, but I thought she was mean.

Mary abandoned him to attend to another patient. In SCU, there were eight or nine spaces just like Dad's. Each nurse watched over two patients. Mary hustled into the next room, glanced at the monitors, checked vital signs, picked up the catheter bag, read levels on saline solutions, and plumped up the pillow. A bigger picture started to unfold for me, and my criticism of her relaxed a bit.

I scanned SCU, all its patients hovering at the edge of life. For a few moments, I studied the long central nurses' and doctors' station, where men and women in uniforms busily reviewed charts and discussed care plans. Behind that thick desk was a room tucked away, where someone read a monitor that monitors the other monitors. I might have suspected a sense of bustle and urgency, but there was calm. Competent professionals filled this space. I surmised that the Special Care Unit must require a special kind of worker.

When Mary spotted me outside Dad's room, peeking in on him as he slept, she brusquely squared off with me, confronted me straight in the eye, and spouted, "Ya?"

Again, I boiled. I wanted to shout, *What do you mean, 'ya?
I'm here to see how my father's doing. Don't you know that, Mary?
I want you to tell me what kind of night he had, MARY! I want to
know if he's still on the critical list. What do you mean, 'ya?'*

I wished I'd been the golf official declaring the ruling, "Mary,
your shot is out of bounds. There will be a penalty."

And then I remembered this very man—whose life I was
here to honor—had taught me a lesson or two. When unpleasant events happened, or stressful situations arose, before any
reaction, Dad always made an assessment, "In twenty years, how
important will this be?"

I had made Mary, R.N., the enemy; but she and I both wanted
one thing—Dad's recovery. We were both motivated by the
same quest. I could, in what appeared to be a cold interaction,
practice warmth.

Dad had also taught me about respect. "You know, you have
to value your opponent. You don't really play against your ri-
val, anyway. You go out there and you play your own best game.
You don't play against someone else. You play the course; the
course is your competitor. If I'm mad at another competitor, or
afraid, it can only defeat my purpose. So you have to stay focused on what's right, and not get thrown off by whatever any
other player does. Any other contender can hit a great shot or
a terrible shot, can be talking to you or swearing, can even be
throwing clubs; none of it matters. What matters is that you
get your own job done, and you do what's best."

The course of Dad's recovery, or perhaps my own present
mind state, was the challenger, not Mary. Mary was just another player. We were playing the same course. Echoing Dad's
words about respect on the links, I recalled a quote: "one way
to destroy an enemy is to make her a friend."

That reminder led me to approach Mary, "I just want to tell

you how hard I see you're working here. It must be really difficult and often thankless to do nursing for such sick patients. I
could never do what you do. I see how you care for people, and
I want you to know that my family really appreciates all the
attention you're giving to my dad."

Mary smiled for the first time. She replied, "Gee, thanks,
let's go see how he's doing."

Then, as if confirming our common goal, she pulled back
his curtain, glanced at the monitors, checked his vital signs,
picked up the catheter bag, read levels on saline solutions, and
plumped his pillow.

At 6:45 a.m., I left the Medical Center, and drove home for
an hour or so of more restful sleep. I returned at 8:30, planning
to meet Vicki, Ann and Mom. The nursing staff had shifted at
7:00 a.m. What did this new tag say? Barbara, Bobbie? Oh, maybe
Betty—Betty was on duty for Dad. The instant I arrived, Betty
flew out of another patient's room, to accost me in an admon-
ishing tone. "Two of your brothers have already come and
gone."

She described them and I nodded, "Dave and Mark."

Next she rushed over to me, grabbed my shoulder, turned
me away from Dad, shook her right index finger at me, and
scolded, "You can't do this. You have to leave him alone. There
are too many of you. You have to stop coming in here. He needs
rest. He can't be entertaining people all the time."

Again anger and resentment flared up in me as initial reflex
reactions, but, more quickly this time, our mutually important
purpose came to mind. I regrouped and responded, "Oh, thanks
for telling me. There really are a lot of us. Seven. I know most
of them are already on their way in. Could I use this phone? If I
don't call now, you'll have to reroute people all day long."

Like Mary, Betty softened, "Well, it's not that you can't come in…just not all at once, and the visits can only be a minute or so. Not all seven on the same day—two a day. Make a schedule."

In order to stop anyone who might still be at home, I phoned immediately. Vicki turned the corner just as I began.

Betty seemed bossy but caring, tough but with Dad's best interest in mind, a no-nonsense get-it-done kind of person. I liked her. After I hustled through the calls, I asked Betty, "Well, I know my mother will want to come in, so that means only one other, right? Only immediate family, and only one a day besides Mom, right? I really respect what you're doing here and I want to make sure I get back to everyone and tell them the right thing."

Betty let go of my shoulder, and Betty, Vicki, and I turned toward Dad. We stole a look. His condition, his position, his breathing were unchanged. "Well," she reconsidered, "your mother can be here anytime. In fact, she can be here all day if she wants, as long as she just sits next to him, so he can see her if he wakes up. No talking."

Then she winked at me, "You understand the need for quiet, don't you? He just can't be using up his energy chatting all day."

She continued, "He had a pretty stable night. We went in a few times to pound on his back, trying to get him to cough in order to prevent pneumonia. He's still nauseous, and won't eat, but we're trying to give him Jell-O-type food. He does seem to have a dry mouth, so we serve him ice and sips of water when he wants them. Managing and adjusting meds is what we'll do here for the next couple of days."

Vic and I took our brief one-minute turns. No speaking allowed. Transmitting as I had the night before, I silently sent him Betty's report. "Dad, it's Sue. I love you. You're doin' fine. You've been taken off a couple of IVs. That's a great sign. It's also a good sign that you recognized all of us yesterday. I'm here, Dad, I know you know that, and I also know neither you nor I can talk right now, so I'll see ya' later."

Vic and I conversed with Betty. "Well, we reached all the kids by phone, but our dad is a pretty popular man, and who knows who might show up. I'm glad you're the kind of person who can speak your mind, because you might have to turn people away until your blue in the face."

"I had that sense about him," Betty laughed. "Don't worry about me. By the way, here's the SCU phone number. Any of you can call me any time to see how your father's doing, and pretty soon he'll be able to have more company. Seven kids, huh? That's pretty amazing. Thanks again for being so considerate."

Having completed a tough round, Vicki and I walked out, arms around each other's shoulders.

✑

By 8:45 a.m., I was aware of much advice: from Whitman—to be "... respectful by habit, constantly honoring the worthy..." and from Dad—"You go out there and you play your own best game. You don't play against someone else. You play the course. The course is your challenger."

Finally, I could embrace both the immediate and the larger implications of Betty's important question, "You understand the need for quiet, don't you?"

TWELVE

WEATHERING HAZARDS

Have you ever noticed what golf spells backwards?
Al Boliska

Monday, June 28, 1999 ✒ Third postoperative day

Golf course architects build courses to create tests for the players. Clubs hire Robert Trent Jones or Donald Ross to plan narrow tree-lined fairways, or a tiny target of a sand-trap-lined green. There are sharp dog legs to the left and blind dog legs to the right. Some holes are long par fives, others are straight up-hill with water hazards all around. The rough is everywhere, and there may be cliffs or rocks to avoid. "It's the course," Dad believes, "that separates the winners from the average player."

Sometimes on courses, there are also temporary hazards, perhaps from a storm's washout, or a sink hole in the middle of the fairway. The course maintenance crews draw thick white lines around these "Ground Under Repair" (GUR) spots. The Rules of Golf state that the ball is in play if it lands in a bunker or on a hill. The ball must be played as it lies, but if the ball lands in a GUR, inside the white lines, there is relief. A player may take a free lift out.

But life is not as fair as the Rules of Golf. Wouldn't it have been wonderful if we could have drawn a big white line around this cardiac event to get a free lift out? We wanted relief. There was none.

❀

Writing provides some reprieve for me, an act of hope, of discovering my feelings, and of connecting with myself and others. Since Dad's admission to the hospital more than a week before, I had sent letters, thank you notes, cards and e-mails. Having received many responses, I felt supported by a broad collective, a big net holding me. This reaching out and this being touched back cracked open my heart. I had not felt alone with the aches and longings. This day I sent the following e-mail message to cousins, aunts, uncles, siblings and some friends:

Hi everyone, Rough day today. Mom and I saw Dad at about noon and he looked much worse: withered, old, wrenching with discomfort, and extremely nauseous. He was on his side waiting to vomit into a little plastic tray that was next to his head. His chest heaved with labored breathing. His voice was barely audible, and he was reattached to some intravenous lines from which he had been disconnected yesterday. An echocardiogram had been ordered, with no results yet. The possibility of getting a pacemaker to his heart was discussed, for he is not responding the way the cardiac team would like as they try to wean him from the I.V.s. His heart rate/ pulse rate plummeted. His blood pressure dropped again today. He's getting discouraged, and doesn't feel very good.

The doctor visited and told him he was doing fine. I asked him, "Dad, do you believe him?"

"No!"

His sister, Anita and her husband, Paul, came by. Anita comforted, "Hey Ray, you look great."

Giving Dad a little poke, Paul chuckled, "No, you don't. Actually, Ray, you look like hell."

"That's more like it," Dad groaned.

A word or two is all he can muster, so Mom and I went to the waiting room to make some calls, and then to the cafeteria. It was not easy. Our bodies were tense. Neither of us had much of an appetite, especially Mom, who was trying, but choking down each bite of her tuna sandwich. I showed her the newly-renovated chapel, where we spent a few moments together—in silence, in our kind of prayer, I suppose—then we returned to SCU.

We heard news that was a bit more hopeful, because the nurse told us what the staff was pleased about: He can talk. He recognizes us. He tolerated a couple of bites of food. He's off the respirator. He's generating a little urine."

Mom asked, "Is he off the critical list?"

"Right now he's stable," was the solemn reply. My stomach landed in my throat.

I wanted to hear, "Yes."

"What we all need," instructed the physicians' assistant (PA), "is patience. He's in a rut right now, and we're all working to get him out, then maybe he'll be moved to the Cardiac Intensive Care Unit (CICU). Usually people go from SCU to the cardiac rehab floor, but it's a big puzzle with him, and we need time to put all the pieces together. He can't go to CICU until many of these special cardiac meds can be reduced and until he can take pills rather than be hooked to I.V.s."

While we were at lunch, they had, indeed, used a hand-held pacemaker to see if they could quicken his heart. They had also disconnected the pain narcotic I.V. thinking that drug might be responsible for so much nausea.

"He's 76," the PA reported, as if we'd forgotten.

"His heart was in bad shape, don't forget," added the nurse.

"Remember, if he had waited another week, he never would have made it. That's how sick he is."

"He had a lot of surgery," we were reminded.

"Patience," the doctors prescribed.

A lot of people are asking how Mom is doing. Better than anyone would have predicted, given the severity of his condition. One of my friends just sent me a quote from Eleanor Roosevelt, which definitely applies to Mom:

"Women are like tea bags. You never know how strong they are until they get into hot water."

When Mom told one of their friends that Dad had had seven arteries repaired, they both laughed together with the realization that, "this man has been breaking records all his life, so this shouldn't surprise anyone."

So, you know, I was remembering his life accomplishments— not to mention his fathering seven kids! He leads the country in club titles at one club (32), and in overall (47) club championships. He has six Maine Amateur titles, and was runner-up five other years. He is the only player to win the Maine High School Championship, Maine Junior and the Maine Amateur in the same year. While he was a student at Bowdoin College, he was both the Maine and the New England Intercollegiate Champion. Now he also has won three New England Senior Amateur titles and a dozen or so Maine Senior wins. He won his first club championship at age 14, and the span of 56 yeas between his first and last wins is two years short of another national record. He's been playing on the Maine Tri-State Amateur Team for 50 years. He's been inducted into both the Maine Sports Hall of Fame and the Maine Golf Hall of Fame. A 1993 article about Dad in *Maine Golf Magazine* ends with these words: "His handicap has varied only slightly, from one to 'plus one' (a stroke better than par) during the last 40 years. That kind of performance may also make Ray Lebel Maine's cham-

pion of consistency."

I notice I relax and soften if I can see the big picture. Sometimes, it feels more like we need to buckle our seat belts and feel the emotional roller coaster, one moment at a time, one bit of news at a time. Fear, hope...sadness, joy...anticipation, relief... All seven of us, and of course Mom, have our own individual and different ways of dealing with all of this.

I'm sure some of you are aware: Today is their 51st wedding anniversary. Dad knew that, or he remembered that Dave had told him yesterday. Dad remembered to say "Happy Anniversary" to Mom first thing today. In fact, last night Ann visited Dad briefly, and he wanted her to do him a favor. "Ann, go into my bag and find a little note. I want you to take it to Mom tonight."

Confused, Ann explained to him, "Dad, Mom will be in early tomorrow. You can give it to her yourself then."

"No," he insisted. "I want her to have this tonight." Like stretching and warming up on the range to get a good swing before stepping up to the first tee, Dad's way to prepare for this round was to make sure Mom had his note on their actual anniversary day.

So, at 9:00 p.m., Ann delivered a handwritten note from Dad at the Maine Medical Center to Mom at home:

"Dear Jeanne,

Thank you for 51 happy years. Love, Ray."

Writing was his final act Friday morning before going into surgery at 8:00 am. He called Mom at 6:30. They talked for a few minutes. He composed the note, and tucked it in his bag. Then the operating room staff came to get him.

Dear folks, Dad is so appreciative of all your cards to him and calls to Mom. Family and friends mean a lot to him. He can't have visitors right now. Only immediate family, only one at a time, and only literally for a minute—a quick kiss and good-bye. I know some of you have already tried to see him, and were turned away by the *staff. We all wish it were different…maybe soon.*

Thank you all for your concerns. Thanks for "listening." As you can imagine, it helps me to write this, makes it all more manageable. The essence of this is that it is so challenging. Yet, feelings of hopelessness and helplessness abate a bit by writing, and by knowing all kinds of people are pulling for him.

Stay tuned. Love to you all, Sue

☙

Whoever was the Grand Architect of this course we found ourselves playing had plans, rules and obstacles for us that we did not fully comprehend. There were no lifts from the rough spots, no smooth ride in a comfortable cart. As on any golf course, there were storms, rain, wind, and strong gales. We did not understand the topography of the land in this crisis, and our game was getting away from us.

Patience, the doctors prescribed. Patience had been one of Dad's best weapons on the golf course. His strong mental focus over the play of a two or three-day tournament wore down even the "young kids," he called them. As his drives lost distance, his eyes dimmed in sharpness, and his arms and legs lost strength over the years; he nevertheless could stay the course, making pars, making birdies. Those who might prevail over him in one-day events marveled at how tough he was over an extended contest. Physically, with aging, the game gets more challenging, yet this game is won mentally, hanging in over an extended ordeal. Although there was no free lift out, we would take a page from the *Ray Lebel Rule Book*. Since we had no strategy of our own, we would adopt his, and practice patience over the long haul.

THIRTEEN

DYING IN EVERYDAY LIFE

For those who seek to understand it, death is a highly creative force. The highest spiritual values of life can originate from the thought and study of death.

Elisabeth Kubler-Ross

Tuesday, June 29, 1999

For the first time with real conviction, I began to entertain the possibility of Dad's imminent death. When Mom and I peered in on him from the entryway to his room, she gripped my arm, and gasped, "Oh, my God, Susan, he looks terrible. I'm really worried about him."

Later, Ann visited Dad, when it was announced that, within minutes, he would be moved to the Cardiac Intensive Care Unit. Incredulous, Ann reported that he looked "really awful...he was totally out of it." In the elevator to CICU, she was concerned enough to give Dad a pep talk about "fighting."

Mike saw him for the first time since surgery, and related

afterward, "It was kind of rough…very tough, actually, to see him like that."

Returning home from a trip to the hospital, Vicki uttered to her husband, "I think we're losing him."

As my fear crescendoed, and weariness from this lengthy vigil set in, I continued to send daily e-mail "updates" to cousins and friends. This day I repeated much of yesterday's news, and added "…moved to CICU, still nauseous—pancreas inflamed…"

Richard Herman, M.D., friend and trustworthy support, answered, "I'm sure, as a nonmedical person, if you've never seen the normal pattern for a man his age who's been through so much, it would be difficult for you to assess how your father is doing."

True. I would learn only later that the third day can be the worst. For that moment, I was convinced that my father was dying.

All week, I had been terrified of the prospect of his passing. I sensed a shift from doubt to certainty, and an inner dialogue took shape. "Instead of rejecting this dread," it began, "could I open to it consciously? What would it be like if I softened around the whole idea? What would happen if I worked to dwell in death's probability? How would acceptance feel? How different from my usual frantic stance would it be to embrace the end of life?"

The fact that I had been denying death's arrival now triggered an ironic chuckle. The interior questioning continued. "As human beings, aren't we the only species that is conscious of our own deaths? And isn't it curious, that this one actuality brings disbelief? How is that we do not understand that death will be everyone's fate—including our own? I, too, am guilty of 'It won't happen to me.' Isn't it interesting how we rail against the only sure thing?"

This was a dilemma. This gnawing anxiety had kept me tight, awake nights and busy all week, but I hadn't been willing to admit it. Now I was creeping in closer to the truth. For sure, there was no way to grieve "correctly," but I needed some help with my refusal to look at this unwanted outcome. So I did what I often do when I feel stuck. I consulted my husband, Jon.

Jon's philosophy is, "Life is full of suffering. So what? We can be happy anyway."

Jon is emotionally steady, with mountain-like solidity. For a quarter of a century now, I had counted on him for the voice of reason.

"Jon," I initiated a dinner conversation. "You wouldn't believe how he looked today. It was so sad to see him; my Dad, my hero. Mom is worried that he's given up. It would be hard to fight, I imagine. You remember that golf ball I gave him the other day? Well, today I put in his hands again, and said, trying to be funny and encouraging, 'Hey Dad, you can use this to imagine yourself back on the golf course.' And he just groaned, 'I could care less.' That's not like him, not to care about golf."

Jon leaned back, preparing to say something. He stroked his moustache, reflecting. Taking a few considered breaths he offered, "You know, I've been considering this. Don't you think all our wishes for him to survive are not for him, but for us? You know, we want him here because we want him around, but it's kind of selfish. He can't really live like this, I mean in the sense of having a life. So, for him, it's better, maybe, that he dies if he has to. This probably sounds weird. Don't get me wrong. I want him to pull through as much as you do. It's just that, while we're saying we're worried about Dad, we're actually worried about ourselves. It's just our egos that don't believe they can survive although of course they will."

Mike, too, who has been preparing for years for the day when

Dad will no longer be here, also advised me, "Sue, it's better to get used to this over time. Statistically, parents die before their kids."

More reality therapy came to me from Dr. Patch Adams, played by Robin Williams in the movie. In an impassioned speech, Patch challenged doctors and medical students to look beyond dying to a fuller appreciation of life. He delivered the line:

"What's wrong with death?"

I decided to practice. My mind devised preparatory experiments in dying. If Dad was going to leave us, I would learn to let go. I would be in training for dying in little ways, so the real end wouldn't hit like a crash course. It felt artificial, silly and contrived. I was perhaps playing at death lightly in order to take the smallest step to the edge of the cliff.

In bed, Jon and I lay next to each other, our bodies spooned together. Every time, an inevitable moment arose when one of us fell away from the other as we drifted into sleep. Only moments before touching my shoulder, his arm dropped. "Oh, man, I hate this part," I complained. "It's like death. You're here next to me one minute. Then—poof! You're gone."

We were like children giggling. Inwardly, I pretended to ready myself for that eventual adult someday when one of us would be alone. All by myself, I rolled away from him. I worked to feel this loss. Deliberately, I put myself in the yoga position called the "corpse pose;" dead to the concerns of the world. On my back, with hands facing up, palms falling away, legs and feet open and relaxed outward, I took a few conscious breaths. As I felt the breath move the body, I noticed the exhale as the breath of release. This was merely a mini-death. I imagined our first breath in life as a gasping in-breath, our last a sighing out-breath. Exhaling, no following inhale … death. At the end of the exhale…. nothing. Right after my exhalation, before the inhalation began, I experienced a gap, a void. With Jon sound asleep now, I experienced this emptiness, that moment of suspension. It felt ridiculous and important at the same time. I was seeking friendship, if not peace, with death, trying to acknowledge my own long-denied mortality. Perhaps working purposefully toward calm acceptance of nothingness might help me release the grasping I'd felt this week. If I could be present to every breath's release, I wondered if I would more easily see that death is part of life.

I had grieved losses before—of three grandparents, of a beloved aunt, of alcohol, of over-exercising, of obsessing about my weight, of the need to get all A's. At these times, both great and small, the illusion of invincibility was crushed and I survived. I kept breathing. With each inhale, I felt Jon's availability. On each exhale, I completely let go. I was not working with specifics—not Jon's dying, or Dad's dying, or my dying. Rather, I directed my attention to the universal death.

Was I comfortable with the idea of Dad's passing? No. Thoughts I wished I weren't having flooded my mind. Unpleasant feelings filled in the gap. Then in this minuscule dose of facing death, I regained the courage to face life. As I softened to the hard reality of death, a new awareness was born: whatever happens, I could trust myself to grieve and recover. Yes, I wanted Dad around. If he died, I would have profound sorrow. Cry. Wrench in pain. Eventually, I would be okay.

I imagined death was with me this day, and the image changed my priorities. Golfers have all sorts of funny lines about players dying on the course, while no one pays attention and the game goes on. "Hit the ball, drag the body."

Although I knew my inner game was fantasy, I could not laugh today at dead golfer jokes. Spiritual teachers, too, like to tease, "The trouble with you is you think you have time." With this ever-so-slight crack in my wall of denial, I realized that I did not, or may not, have the luxury of many more days. If today had been my last, or Jon's last, or Dad's last (which, of course, it might have been), I would want to tell my loved ones how I feel. If today's were my final actions, then I would go to Mom. If these hours are all we had, I would spend them with my family in the hospital. Life is precious. Life is sacred. Every moment matters.

FOURTEEN

EMBRACING MYSTERY

Whenever we penetrate the heart of things, we always find a mystery. Life and all that goes with it is unfathomable. Knowledge of life is recognition of the mysterious.

Albert Schweitzer

Wednesday, June 30, 1999

The fourteenth day. I fell asleep repeating, again and again, "Two weeks. It's been two weeks. Fourteen days. How long will this last?"   "Fourteen" became the mantra and the induction as I dozed off into this dream:

ⓖ

I am a teenager again, and I stand, across the suburban street from where we live, on the back nine of the Portland Country Club. Waites Landing abuts the thirteenth green, the fourteenth hole and the fifteenth tee, and I take a tiny khaki-colored canvas bag filled with six or seven clubs to play those three holes often. All by myself, because I never feel good enough to play with anyone else, I go round and round. I go for fun and stress relief, not to play golf, really, but to be outside, to get some sun and a little exercise. Sometimes I start on fifteen, then play thirteen, then fourteen. Round and round.

But fourteen is my favorite, because it's short. An easy par three with colorful flower beds around the hilly green, the fourteenth hole sports trimmed bushes between the green and the fifteenth tee. I can see the faint edges of my house for the whole length of play, as the fourteenth fairway runs parallel to Waites Landing. I can sometimes save par on fourteen. I like fourteen because it is a link, a break between the long thirteenth and the even longer fifteenth. Sometimes I hit the tee shot, play out the hole, then walk back to the fourteenth tee and play that same hole again. I feel like a golfer there.

So here I am in this dream, on fourteen, praying as I always do, that I will not cross paths with Dad and his tournament-level, champion-quality, golfer-type buddies. Yet here they are, holing out on thirteen, and waiting for me to tee off on fourteen. I dread their watching me or seeing my swing. So I cry, "Dad, I can't play this game like you do. I need your help."

He laughs, looks at Al, Frank, and Mike, and commiserates, "I cannot stay alive in this game today either, so maybe I can give you a lesson. It'll help both of us."

He stands behind me, his belly against my back, and patiently wraps his hands—those strong, hairy, stout, accurate-surgeon, horn-playing, golfer hands—over my unsteady teenage ones on the grip. "Here," he comforts, "let's help each other."

✿

Mom and I still shook from yesterday's experience of seeing Dad so close to death. We were cautious and squeamish as we departed the echoing ninth floor elevator and began our walk on the speckled shiny brown and white tile floor, down the wide, sterile hospital corridor. The bustling hall was filled with the soft voices of nurses and technicians comforting patients as they pushed beds around corners. On our way to the Cardiac Intensive Care Unit, we passed a small waiting area on our left. In upright wooden-backed chairs with plastic avocado-colored seats, anxious visitors paced back and forth in this narrow space. Others sat, reading *The Portland Press Herald* or watching the *Today Show* on the tiny wall-mounted television.

There were flurries of activity on this "heart floor." Today the busy-ness and noise had an order which I had not, as yet, detected. People were doing what they must do, nurses serving patients, who practiced patience while waiting for their doctors who read charts and adjusted medications. Visiting families witnessed it all, came and went, offered love. There was rightness in the way things were. Yesterday I had only been aware of the messiness, the discord. Now I sensed the vital force holding it all. Until now, my mind had been blinded by its own chaos. Embracing the underlying calm in this surface turbulence, I could more easily accept this human mystery, and Dad's questionable destiny. Thankfully, I was learning to be in the bunker and figuring out how to play my way out.

With new courage, I approached Dad's room with Mom. Punching the round silver knob which is the automatic opener for the door to CICU, I marched ahead to see Dad. Before the first step landed, Mom tugged at my untucked t-shirt, and whispered, "Oh, God, I hope he looks better than he did yesterday."

We turned the final corner. We braced ourselves. We peeked in. Again, Mom yanked my arm, and gasped, "Oh, my God! Look at him!" There sat the Dad I had always known.

In his chair.

Upright.

Blue cotton robe, white nylon knee socks covering his scarred legs, hospital-issued blue paper slippers.

Glasses on his face.

Hands holding cards, slitting open envelopes.

Reading people's handwriting.

He glanced up, spotted us, smiled, and said, "Hi."

He, too, had turned a corner. We talked, a few words. He joked. We conversed, longer sentences. We laughed.

Later, at home, I wrote another e-mail:

"WOW!! The wonders of modern medicine. He's coming around. The roller coaster took us to the edge, woke us up a bit, shook up the family, and the human spirit shines through. Amazing."

A vision kept repeating itself. I saw Dad in CICU until he was more stable, hooked up to many machines, needles, and bags. He was nauseous, suffering many complications. My golf dream haunted me. It had been fourteen days with little break between the surgery and the recovery. Now perhaps we might be granted a reprieve, like on that fourteenth hole. As if standing on the fourteenth tee next to Waites Landing, we began to see the faint outline of home. Hands linked together, we were helping each other finish up the back nine.

The mystery of fourteen kept me from sleeping, and my dad, my tournament-level, champion-quality father, WAS staying alive in this game today.

I got out of bed, and wrote:

MYSTERY

The man I call Dad is back.
What happens to the human spirit when the body is cut wide
    open,
chest invaded,
sternum cracked,
    legs searched for veins,

throat forced to accept tubes,
            neck, wrists, arms, pierced with needles?
...when machines do the breathing and technology does the
    pumping?
Where is my father in this?
I wonder.

And how is that three days after his being inside out,
there is a big decline?
He was gone.
That person we knew and loved
had slumped to a different man,
one seemingly giving up, failing.

Not wanting to accept the ups and downs of this course,
hoping against hope for an uphill,
one-way,
linear,
    straight trajectory
            from this artificial death
                    to vibrant new life,
we clutched.

We do not always get what we want.
The gods teased us with two "steady progress" days,
a few funny words,
a little hand squeeze,
    the emerging of our man.
We wanted more of this.

Yet, on the third day, mystery rules.
A dive into pain,
and nausea,
    and not caring—even for golf.

We struggled to accept things as they were.
Trying to learn patience.
  But we did not understand.

We wanted life the way we expected it.
Even though our illusions of predictability
had been shattered before,
From these depths we nevertheless imagined
long,
slow,
step-by-step,
  sequential improvement,
      one grateful breath at a time.

Silly humans. Wrong again.
We forgot to allow for mystery
and miracles
  and the care and protection of Higher Forces.
We forgot about quantum leaps.
We forgot that, when the personality cannot fight,
  Something Deeper fights for us.
And we forgot how many times Ray Lebel has recovered from
  the rough.
Once again, we were forced to let go our limited preconcep-
  tions

.....................because................

from withered old unrecognizable stranger,
arises Raymond.
Now we open our eyes,
we see Ray.

We recognize his essence,

his watery grayish-green-blue eyes appear,
behind tired lids, for sure,
   his twinkling windows of the soul
              sparkle back at us nevertheless.
Hiding deep inside,
drawing from some mysterious source of strength,
Ray Lebel claims life.

From death's door
to sitting in his chair,
a throne-like statement of victory,
his masterful surgeon's hands now opening mail,
   humor returning to tease nurses about golf,
   joking as he laughs with Mom.
She touches his arm, now growing new hair, and notices
   warmth.
Hand-to-hand,
he is winning the toughest tournament of his life.

There is a place for all seven of us in this.
Each of the seven repaired arteries has one of our names on it.

As Dad is anchor for us in seven different ways,
we are shown through his return
that we are each an important strand in the web of this family.
We feel blessed with a rekindled knowing of this,
a new respect for modern Western medicine,
and especially for the undercurrent of the life force.
He is stepping up to the tee now,
And we all breathe a collective sigh of relief.
He is alive,
not only not dead
   not only surviving and gasping for each breath,
       but swinging.

Now it's on to addressing the ball of life.
The vigil has ended.
    The man I call Dad is back.

FIFTEEN

LIGHTENING UP

*The reason the pro tells you to keep your head down
is so you can't see him laughing.*
~Phyllis Diller

Thursday, July 1, 1999

*On the front of a card: Patient: "Oh, doctor, I'm so nervous
about this operation. It's my first one!"*
Surgeon: "Don't worry, it's mine, too!"
On the inside: Rest easy. You're in good hands.

It was only noon, and Dad said he was so exhausted that it felt like nine at night. Dad would remain in the Cardiac Intensive Care Unit until certain cardiac drips could be stopped and his heart started on its own. Today the pacemaker had been discontinued and we were waiting to see how he responded. His voice was weak and scratchy. Although the nausea had subsided, his appetite had not returned. With the help of medication, he had slept well. Though we felt gripped by darkness, a bright energy also spread through the family. Lightheartedness heals. Throughout last week's diagnostic phase and even on the very most intense day of surgery, we kept our sense of humor. There had been long faces, and also some levity. As we visited today—Mom, Mike, Paul and I—we laughed together at the many heartfelt cards he had received:

Cover: Don't think of it as being in the hospital.

Inside: Think of it as a tremendously expensive vacation in an unfashionable resort that just lost its chef.

Get well soon.

⑥

It is well known in scientific literature that the use of humor has direct physiological benefits. Studies show that humor helps the body cope with stress. There is less fatigue, tension, anger, depression and confusion. By now Norman Cousins' *Anatomy of an Illness* is well-read. In this book, he outlined his remission from chronic illness. Crediting his increase in health to his self-treatment with hilarious movies, Cousins labeled the healing power of laughter, "internal jogging." Humor possesses a stress-buffering effect which also enhances immune function. Our use of wit throughout Dad's hospitalization did not bubble up because we knew this research. As paradox, this effervescence sparkled naturally from connecting with the flatness of fear. Coming up close and touching human suffering directly enabled us to tap into a deeper happiness, unruffled by external circumstances. There is joy in being fully human, even when it is difficult. Especially when it is difficult.

⑥

Vicki visited, delivering a huge poster displaying the face of Jack Nicklaus. We hung it on a little pink curtain above a window in Dad's room, clearly visible from his bed. As she unrolled it, and clipped on the pins, Vicki quipped, "Hey, Dad, I figure with the Bear looking over you here, you'll perk up in no time."

⑥

Golf jokes arrived in cards in the mail:

Cover: Don't worry about your operation! Your doctor says that after your surgery, you'll be able to play golf the same as before.

Inside: But other than that, you'll be just fine.

⑥

On Dad's bedside tray was a pink plastic kidney-bean-shaped tub, in case his nausea returned. Next to it was a spirometer, a small device to help Dad learn to breathe deeply, so as to prevent pneumonia. Also on the table was a thirty-year-old photograph of all seven of Dad's children and Mom dated December, 1969. Dad must have been behind the camera. Ann framed the picture in Lucite, and printed on the blue mat, "Come Home Soon! We Love You!" Our clothes were dated, the colors out of style. All four of my brothers had full heads of hair in this picture. Ann was pouting. Teenage Mark was holding young Dave, while Dave giggled, trying to pull free. My hair, as a twenty-year-old, was bleached platinum, highly teased. We were a motley crew.

And there was more fun to offset the medical supplies. A final piece adorned the stand—a bright yellow and green fake daisy plant in an earthen-colored equally fake pot. When pushed, a small button on the side blasted, "HELLLOOO! Good morning! Isn't this a beautiful day?" Next burst forth a shrill shrieking of the "Daisy, Daisy" tune:

Daisy, daisy,
up with the morning dew,
and now it's time
to rise and shine
as I wish a good day to you.

The contrast between the seriousness of the CICU room, —the tubes, the I.V.s and bags, the spirometer, the tray for vomiting, the life-support machines—with the silliness of the family photo and the crazy plant was striking.

⑥

Dad told the story many times of his interview with Dr. Bucknam, an admissions officer at Tufts Dental School. Twenty-something Ray Lebel was nervous, having an introverted personality. He had always been more inclined toward action than words. Since his childhood, Dad had yearned to practice oral surgery, and had trained in the office of his favorite uncle, an oral surgeon in Lewiston, Maine. A short man, young Ray walked into to the admissions office, shook hands with the large man who stood up from behind his huge and impressive desk.

"I have a cottage in Maine. I saw you play at Augusta. I even have ties to your Dad, as my sister was his kindergarten teacher. So, you are a pretty hot golfer, I hear," roared Dr. Bucknam.

Flashes of his own father reminding him not to be cocky rushed through his head. "Well, yes, sir, I enjoy the game."

"So would you rather talk golf, dentistry, or world events?"

Dad was not as conversant about dentistry as Dr. Bucknam, but he had the good sense to know that he probably could out-talk this powerful examiner in the game of golf. Yet he also wondered if this was a trick question. So Dad chuckled, which helped his sturdy shoulders drop a bit. "Well, sir, I certainly would be a lot more comfortable talking about golf."

He had no idea what might happen next, or what this would mean for any possible acceptance. This honest remark from a young would-be dentist was followed by silence and a few tense breaths. "Okay then, let's talk golf."

The interview and golf stories ended twenty minutes later

when Dr. Bucknam said, "Tufts Dental School would like to have you. I knew that when you came in. By the way thanks for the golf tips."

⑥

This day in the Cardiac Intensive Car Unit, Dad remained on the critical list. He had no idea what might happen next, or what it would mean for any possible acceptance to the next level of his care and health. Fifty years after his admissions interview, he was still—always—comfortable talking about golf. Mom, Dad, Vicki, and I began to play with the idea of a special gift for Patti, Dad's competent and compassionate CICU nurse. She was new to the game of golf, and, upon discovering Dad's status as a great golfer, had asked his permission to tell her husband that he was her patient. "Of course," Dad answered. "Have him come in and we can spend hours talking about the game."

Although CICU was quiet, we were rowdy making our plan for Patti and her husband. It would be fun to create a present to show Dad's gratitude for her kind attention—a type of care package filled with items for the game of golf. Mom ran home and created a small bag, colorfully decorated with a pastoral golf scene on the outside. She filled it with driving range golf balls, tees and ball markers. Vicki retrieved a "sleeve" of brand new balls, three balls in one package. I bought two special women's balls, and we all returned to the hospital. As a gag, Dad decided to autograph the new balls with a purple Sharpee laundry pen; the sleeve of three for her husband; the two women's balls for Patti. With not quite full-out fanfare, he presented the package to Patti. Her face lit up. Her wide smile and raised eyebrows showed her surprise and delight. Her legs buckled; her knees bent as if to fall back with gratitude. Then she discovered the signed balls. "Wow, this is great. I can't wait to show my husband."

Winking at her, Dad joked, "Now, Patti, don't lose those balls in the woods because they have my name on them."

We left the hospital that day, no different from other days, really. Dad's health was still wavering. He could not yet be moved to the cardiac rehabilitation floor. In the middle of this threatening situation, we were all—Dad included—also frolicking. We experienced what the scientists had proven; with some lightening up, we encountered joy, gained optimism, developed hope, and touched playfulness. Having offered him support, and having shared in mutual jesting, we walked out. I remembered a tease he threw out one day when he read a story in Golf Digest about himself years ago. Until he saw it in print, he had not really been aware of his string of forty-seven golf club championship victories and the fact that he held so many national records. All he offered was, "I guess my longevity was pretty good."

For the first time this week, we were counting on that longevity. With smiles on our faces, we waved "good-bye," and left Dad laughing at the cards:

Cover: Congratulations on the successful completion of your surgical procedure.

Inside: Doesn't that sound better than "Going under the knife and living to tell about it?"

...Hope you're all better soon.

SIXTEEN

REVEALING TRUE NATURE

If I were in a position to hire people, I'd ask them to play golf with me. In eighteen holes, I could learn a lot about them. Do they lie? Do they cheat? How do they react to victory or defeat?
Ray Lebel

Friday, July 2, 1999

All I.V.s and tubes had been removed, and machines discontinued. His breathing was deeper; there were no more sounds of rattling and crackling in his lungs.

Nurses and doctors had commented these past two weeks about the character of this man. Warren Alpern, one of Dad's cardiologists, last week whispered to me, "Your father has strong protoplasm, and in this business, that's important."

I wanted clarification. "You mean life energy, that vitalizing force?"

Without hesitation, Dr. Alpern answered, "That's exactly what I mean."

๑

John Love, Dad's chief cardiologist at Maine Medical Center, revealed, "Right from the start, I've been confident that your father would make it through, because, other than his heart, he's a very strong man."

❀

Right before Dad left CICU, I motioned Patti aside in the hall and asked, "How are his spirits…for real, Patti? You know, he could be putting on a good front for us, but I want to know, how is he really?"

She beamed, "Oh wonderful! What a great man. He's interested in life. He's talking about what he'll do after he leaves here. He brags about his family. He really cares about people. He's interested in us, and asks questions about our lives. Everyone who goes into his room says the same thing."

❀

Dad's protoplasm, his inner strength, and his regard for people reminded me of an old story about human personality. *A veteran was trying to teach a young student the concept of "true nature," of how "we are who we are." The mentor asked the pupil, "What do you get when you squeeze an orange?"*

"Orange juice?" was the quizzical reply.

"Right. What if a kind mother squeezes the orange, what will come out?"

"Orange juice."

"Right. What if an angry father squeezes the orange, do you still get orange juice?"

"Yes, orange juice."

"Right. What do you get when you squeeze a lemon?" The lesson continued.

"Lemon juice?"

"Yes."

The trainee was beginning to catch on, "I get it. It doesn't mat-

ter who or what does the squeezing. If you squeeze a lemon, you'll always get lemon juice."

"So, if you squeeze an orange, will you ever get lemon juice?"

"No," replied the youngster.

"If you squeeze a lemon, will you ever get orange juice?"

"No," the game was becoming exasperating. "If you squeeze a lemon, you'll get lemon. If you squeeze an orange, you'll get orange. Period!"

"So it is with our true nature," the Master explained. "People are who they are, whether they are being squeezed by stress and misfortune or whether life is going along easily and pleasantly. We often try to blame the situation or another person for our reactions, but when people get squeezed, who they really are comes to the surface. Especially under pressure, our inner essence arises. So, then, how one lives is reflected in how one goes through difficulties. How else could it be? If there is no anger inside, then there cannot be any anger under pressure. If anger does surface, then it means that it's been inside the whole time. The onset of anger has little to do with the situation. On the other hand, if a person is filled with kindness, then kindness will also materialize during stress."

©

Through these present difficulties, we noticed the true expression of Dad's essence. Last week, before surgery, when Vicki was in California, she called him every day. He told her not to worry, then began asking her how she liked the golf courses, and how she and her husband were playing. Instead of focusing on what was wrong with himself, Dad asked her, "how's your game?"

He then filled Vicki with golf advice and wisdom.

Certainly, Mike experienced Dad's compassion upon returning from Hawaii. Dad was more interested in Maui than his own symptoms and had less self-concern and more excitement about Mike's enjoyment of the trip.

With obvious discomfort, Dad greeted Mike, "Hey Mike, how was Hawaii?"

Mike tried to ask, "Hey Dad, how are *you?*"

But Dad left no room for talk of his surgery and his pain, diverting the attention back to the golf courses in Hawaii. Mike assumed it would be normal for Dad to tell the story of how he had been stationed near there in the Pacific Theater during World War II, a fighter pilot on the escort carrier, the *Suwannee*. Dad did not talk about himself. Rather, he asked, "What's up with you?"

Today Dad commented on how many thoughtful cards he had received and how many friends and family members had called Mom. He was particularly touched by the well-wishes of people whom he would never expect to reach out, whom he hardly knew. He made a mental note to himself and asked Mom, "Jeanne, can you write down the names of all the people who have contacted me? I want to write to each of them and thank them. It's just remarkable how great people have been."

When I arrived, he lay in bed, eyes closed, earphones on, head bopping to music. I touched his arm and he declares, "Oh, hi, Sue. I was just sitting here thinking of how I could help people. You know, they said I probably had two or three silent heart attacks over the past few months and I never knew it. Now that the doctors tell me what they feel like, I think I know right when they were. I remember that time with Vic on the golf course, when I was having a hard time catching my breath. Maybe I should go on the road and speak about that, so it doesn't have to happen to other people."

Mom entered with Anita who carried presents for Dad. One was a small package of blank colorful thank you cards. He smiled, "Oh, this is great. I want to write to everyone."

There were also four gold foil-wrapped boxes of locally-made chocolates, to be distributed in appreciation from Mom and Dad to the staffs on each of the four floors where Dad had been a patient. Again, Dad remarked, "Oh, great. I've been wondering what I could do for all these incredible doctors and nurses."

Anita also brought a gift box of chocolates for Dad to keep in his hospital room, to offer to his MMC guests. With thoughts of Dad not having any appetite, and having difficulty eating Jell-O and applesauce, we laughed at the idea of an opened box of chocolates on his bed stand. Using her fingernail to slit the plastic outer wrap, Anita then uncovered the box to eat the first one. Amused at the irony of Dad struggling to eat his Cheerios at 10:00 a.m., while we ate candy, we wondered about chocolate and junk food at a time like this.

"Hey, I heard that there are feel-good chemicals and healing hormones in chocolate. What do you think?"

"Actually, chocolate is a vegetable. It grows from the ground, you know."

"Do you think if *we* eat these chocolates, that *Dad* will get better?"

⑥

Next, Dad opened a journal from Anita, who insisted, "Ray, you have to write about this experience."

"No, I don't. Susan is."

More jesting. More fun.

Just then the wife of the man in the next bed popped up angrily from her chair and marched directly to our side of the room. "Could you all be quiet? I'm happy that you're happy, but my husband has just had two-way by-pass surgery, is very sick and needs to be silent."

We hushed, and Dad told us that this roommate spent last night yelling for the nurse, rather than using the call button.

He made so much noise that he continually interrupted Dad's sleep. There was no silence and no rest for Dad. I asked him, "Did you say anything to him?"

"No, he was having a hard time. It wouldn't have been very kind of me to be demanding."

❻

Squeezed by a loud roommate, Dad was kind. Challenged by seven-way coronary by-pass surgery, he considered the needs of others. His most fundamental human impulse was an open heart. As the old teacher might predict, when circumstances squeezed Ray Lebel, what emerged was Ray Lebel. This was the same man who once said to me, "You know, lots of guys get really out of control on the golf course. In all the years I've played major and minor tournaments, I never have. One friend said to me a while back, 'You know, Ray, I've been playing golf with you for fifty years, and I've never seen you throw a club.' I said, 'And you know what? You never will.'"

Dad's essence had not been lost on us. By his touching us, we then touched our own children, coworkers, friends, and strangers in the grocery store. From Mom and Dad, through the seven of us, there were then fourteen grandchildren, and six great-grandchildren. Hear Dad now brought forth in Dave's words:

Dad,
I just want to take the time to say I love you,
and I'm so thankful you found the strength to pull through,
because without you, I don't know what we'd all do.
You see, you're the only one who could ever fill up your shoes.

You've always been the one we all look up to.
I wish I could take back all the bad times I put you through.

Not a day goes by when I don't think about you.
So I want to take the time to say I love you.

I just want to take the time to say thank you
for being there every time we all needed you.
Your example is not an easy one to live up to.
Just want you to know that I will always try to,
and I'm so grateful that you're still here to talk to.

You've never once put yourself before me.
I'm sorry it took so long for me to see.
I think you may have made it all too easy.
I realize now that nothing comes free.

And I just want to take the time to say thank you.

Love, Dave

SEVENTEEN

COMING HOME, BEGINNING AGAIN

What we call the beginning is often the end.
And to make an end is to make a beginning.
The end is where we start from.
T.S. Elliot

Saturday, July 3, 1999

For a day and a half on the cardiac rehabilitation floor, Dad had eaten small amounts of food. Several times each day, he walked a few steps. Of course, we all asked the question, "When will he be discharged?"

Of course, the response was, "We never know. It depends on all kinds of variables."

With that answer, we were all—Dad included—constantly reminded of the precautions necessary to keep him alive. Every instant, human vulnerability presented itself. Yesterday, Dr. Love teased us with, "Maybe tomorrow. We'll monitor what happens with his blood pressure. Let's see what kind of day he has."

We didn't really know exactly what he meant, so we experienced the present moment anxiety while holding out hope for the future wellness. There was less light in this general-wing room than in the large-windowed CICU cubicles. In CICU the staffed spoke in hushed tones. Here, as I sat next to Dad, who lay drugged and shivering, I heard the nurses clogs clicking down the hall. Dad's bed was closest to the hallway, and his roommate, who was nearer the window, had drawn his curtain around him, shading Dad. The scent of dirty laundry wafted; more patients on this floor, more activity. I longed to visit Dad in his own cozy den, right off their newly renovated kitchen with the gray and black lighthouse stenciling on the border, and the hot water spigot within easy reach. Both the water and the spilled ginger ale on the portable table next to his mechanical bed were flat and tepid, ice melted long ago, straw bent over the now half-empty plastic cups.

Dad had begun the transition to home—getting in and out of bed, sitting up, hobbling around, shaving, tasting food. For years, on the gold rug in the family room, Dad had kept a putter, a ball, an indoor mat and "hole." Watching TV, he practiced putting. On his way out of the room, he dared a shot or two. All seven of us attempted to play with this in-house green, and inevitably hit a weak ball which never approached the hole. "Never up, never in," was his advice for putting. "You can hit plenty of greens in regulation figures, but if you leave the putts short, you're dead. You need to think about what you're trying to accomplish. You gotta be specific about your target. Pick your line. Go for it. You can't be tentative. You make your mind up. Then you go."

Whether skirmishing to stay alive in a golf tournament, or fighting for his life, Dad was a fierce competitor, with the historical experience, the courage and fervor to hang tough. He never clutched at great championship moments. Nor did he now. These few days post-CICU were for "Phase One," postoperative in-hospital rehabilitation, on Recovery Floor One (R1). Mom entered at 10:00 a.m. or so. Wearing a clean blue and white hospital Johnny, barely lifting his head, cracking open one eye, and keeping his lips mostly closed, Dad mumbled, "Hmmm."

Mom knelt, setting her face next to his. Lifting her hands, she placed them around his closed palm, and brushed his unshaven cheek with a kiss. "Hi, hon. I love you."

He smiled, "I love you, too."

"How're you feeling today?"

"I don't know yet."

She was aware that the protocol for R1 is that he get up, move, and she wondered if he needed to push himself a bit more. Or was he still too weak, and should he relax? She posed a yes/no question, perhaps easier for both of them. "Any word about going home yet?"

The wondering did not plague us with the hopelessness of a few days earlier. With the passing of time, we held more trust in the healing process and considerable faith in his inevitable homecoming.

"Maybe today." Now he pressed his palms into the mattress and raised his upper body to sitting. Letting his frail legs drop over the side of the bed, he pointed out the leg heavily bandaged from the site where the cardiac surgeon borrowed veins.

"Help me up," he lifted his elbow for support.

Dad had his target in mind, and was hitting it hard. He knew what he was trying to accomplish. Never up, never out of here. Not wanting to be on R1 four or five more days, he picked his sight line: getting home as soon as possible. He stood up. He sat in his chair instead of staying in bed. He got dressed. He sucked on morsels of food, though he had no appetite. "You gotta be specific about your target. Go for it. You make your mind up. Then you go."

This morning the announcement came, "Today is the day. You can go home."

The possibility of regaining personal identity commingled with cold feet. Dad could wear his own clothes again and eat home cooked meals; he would also be further from any needed medical care.

Indeed, the end of his hospitalization was yet again another beginning. For two weeks, we had experienced the full roller coaster of human emotion: fear, sadness, anticipation, relief, anger, confusion, joy. Simultaneously we had grounded ourselves in the probability of Dad's healthier days to come, his statistically more-than-likely full recovery and the big picture of his return to the golf course. Today was no different. When I took my emotional pulse, there was fear, joy, confident expectation and caution.

The cardiac event was over for now. The rehabilitation had begun. Making some predictions, the discharge nurse tallied his scorecard.

"He may not feel like eating for a while. You may spend all day cooking his favorite foods, and he'll push it away at the table. His improvements may be slow or they may be big, and some days it may look like there is no progress. You may feel discouraged. He can start walking, and he should, but he may not be happy about it. His spirits may be fine one minute and despondent the next. In a few weeks, the doctor will grant him permission to drive and you may not think he's ready. You'll work hard to make things okay for him. When people come to visit, they won't always ask how the family is doing. Infection may develop. If you notice it, call us right away. An extra beat or beats may show up in his pulse. Make sure you get him right in here if that happens."

This ending was clearly the place from where we would start.

As deeply held assumptions—about trusting the body, about mortality, about the illusion of invincibility—were being challenged, we slowly discovered the value of connecting with others. It began by entering the Maine Medical Center and placing Dad's life in the hands of physicians and nurses whose skill and knowledge helped sustain his existence. Now he would return home and start to expand his life again.

I wrote in my journal:

So we begin. We begin with a new awareness of the universality of human suffering. We begin with a new sense of appreciation for the web of support that has helped us. Mom has held Dad's hand, we have held Mom's hand, and a wide network of friends is holding each of our hands. We are strengthened by these connections. Because of this net of concern which is cast by others, we can begin to trust our own ability to work with our changing emotional states. We begin with gratitude for whatever it is in the human spirit (Grace? Courage? Strength? Integrity?) that grants us the ability to face whatever has been and will be handed us, that stuff we would never predict we could handle. Something in us has been awakened these past two weeks. Today, the day of discharge, we begin again.

(6)

The circumstance of this hospitalization was not like the eighteenth hole of a tournament. "It's over. Congratulations, Dr. Lebel. You won. Now go home and rest."

If you are a golfer, a tournament may end, but the game is never over. Whether he won or not, Dad hit hundreds of balls on the driving range—over and over again, one day after another, evenings after work, and Saturday mornings. As he got older and could not hit the ball so hard or so long, he spent just as many hours chipping and putting. Buckets and buckets of balls.

This hospital discharge is as if Dad has just finished the first stage of Qualifying School. Q School, as it is called, is the Professional Golf Association's Tour Qualifying Tournament, which would-be professional golfers must endure to make the pro circuit. It is grueling, discouraging, and often ends in agony. Tour School is four rounds for Stage One, four rounds for the second stage and six rounds in the final and most difficult stage. It is, perhaps, no coincidence that at least one stage of Q School has been played at Bear Lakes, Dad's home course in West Palm Beach, Florida.

Now Dad, too, was grinding it out, over a multitude of days, getting to the end, with all the anguish of knowing that "one missed putt," one wrong prescription, or one case of pneumonia could disqualify him. This disqualification was not about being able to play professional golf; rather this Q School for Dad is a fight to be "on the right side of the grass," as he dares to joke. Like the putt of the young golfer whose one stroke can make or break his PGA hopes, so Dad's life was hanging on the lip of the cup.

Sometimes golfers go through Tour School several times before they make it to the tour. Some never do. In this first stage, Dad had lost a few holes, met with stormy weather, pulled out of the rough a few times, and missed a putt or two. He had, it seemed, ended up with a decent lie. Yet there was no turning in his score card yet. The practice and the buckets of balls would continue to help, as recovery had only begun. There would be multiple rounds ahead.

It never rains on the golf course because golfers love the game. If it weren't for the rules—that insist that they clear the course during lightning—golfers would play in thundershowers. Now we must play through this weather in our lives. This is bucket work.

EIGHTEEN

DOING THE WORK OF THE HEART

Don't take the attitude, like so many I know, 'Oh, I'm too old to do that.' You're never too old in this game. … If you have keenness and determination, there isn't anything you can't accomplish in this game.

Ben Hogan

August 7, 1999 ⤳ *One month later*

This is the eighteenth chapter, but its story will not be like the eighteenth hole. We went "back to the basics," as Dad advised in golf.

"Remember the fundamentals," Dad taught. "No matter what, keep it simple."

How would I remember the lessons of this game? How would I live now, having experienced what I just experienced? What did I plan to do with my own numbered rounds? Doesn't everyone die eventually and surprisingly? What would it mean to play every moment with the heart of a champion?

⑥

When people saw me, their first question was, "How's your Dad?"

I often replied, "Oh, he's fine. He's coming along."

This was true. Immediately, the inquirer nodded the head, "Oh, great."

I sensed relief in the listener. The "Oh, great" was so quick, so facile. The automaticity relayed the message, "Phew. I heard what I wanted to hear. Now I'm comfortable. Things are okay. All is well."

With the mind's decision that "this is good," any further thought or wrestling with life's perplexity became rendered unnecessary. Discussion closed.

By contrast, there was at least one other way to acknowledge, "How's your Dad?"

"Well, he's having a tough time. Last week he was rushed back to the hospital because of a disturbing and scary arrhythmia. ER workers hooked him to a monitor again for a whole day. His meds are constantly evaluated and sometimes changed. In addition, this week he has an ugly, red, swollen infection like a bad divot on his ankle. So he had to go back to the doctor again. Now he is taking massive doses of antibiotics to fight off any possible staff infection which could kill him."

Often the response which followed resembled, "Oh, that's too bad."

Discussion closed. Or comebacks were often, "Oh, he'll be fine soon. It just takes time."

The categories of "fine" and "not fine" intrigued me. "Fine" is what we want to hear; we can even make "fine" from "not fine." With either response, something in me collapsed. I was left hurt, not heard. I wondered why people ask, "how are things?" if they only expected a one-word answer.

But I needed more. No one would ever ask a golfer, "How was your game today?" and anticipate the answer, "Fine."

Wouldn't the response contain a play-by-play? Would it not

include that topped tee shot on number three, that missed putt on nine? Wouldn't the reply also recount how mad you were at yourself for taking two shots to get out of the thick rough on five, and how proud you were to sink a twenty-footer on twelve? What about chipping away at the whole truth?

Tempted to relate a more complete picture of Dad's reality, I entertained the idea of offering statements of fact with no judgments of good or bad attached. I suspected I might lose the listener:

"He's hitting all the fairways … He got ahead of himself … He's hitting it solid … He hit into the water … He's breathing more easily… He tires quickly … He sleeps better at night … He walked a mile … He has no appetite … He has gained back four pounds of the thirty plus that he lost … He misses the guys at the Club … He's bored and feels lazy sitting around … He's starting to pitch and putt.

You know how he always thought his short game was his weakest? Well, now he recommends clocking in plenty of time on the practice green, so you can pick up around the green what you lose in distance as your long shots get shorter … Next he might try bunker shots…It'll be another few weeks before he can play his first round…

… He's looking forward to moving back to Florida in October … He started the Phase Two Cardiac Rehab Program this week."

My Dad taught me to see the big picture. "In golf, you know, you have to manage the course by seeing the whole thing, from tee to green. You see the shot that's right in front you and, of course, this is the only swing that counts. At the same time, you have to view what's up ahead before you come back to hit the shot."

When he tried to teach me how to swing a club, he always

emphasized, "you have to swing through the ball. You can't stop at the moment of impact. The power comes from executing a swing that follows through. In putting, you stroke through the ball. The follow-through is a most important part."

So it was with Phase Two. He was weak, needed monitoring when he exercised, was learning what to eat to support a healthy heart, how to manage stress. The power of his recovery would be in his follow-through. He couldn't stop at the moment of discharge from the hospital. In these first days at home, the transition was like leaving the comfortable golf lesson with the caring pro, and playing now in competition alone. The doctors and nurses were no longer bedside to coach, and the terrain was hilly with plenty of hazards.

❧

Another journal entry:

He was shocked that his medications cost him $4,000.00 last month ... Yesterday the druggist overcharged him, and in order to apologize, gave him this month's dosage free ... More of the time his spirits are hopeful and positive ... He is peaked, pale, weak, and emaciated ... His heart is working at twenty percent capacity, which is the same as it was before the surgery ... He was told that he feels better only because of his medications; without the double dose of the cardiac stimulant, he would be no better than before the surgery ...

... Saturday he played trumpet at Kristin's (his third oldest grandchild) wedding as he had promised before surgery... He had to wear a sweater vest to take up the slack of his now baggy suit coat, and to keep himself warm.

He gets cold easily. His fingers are skinny, yet still nimble.

His breath was hesitant, but he stood up with Peter Albert's band, blowing his horn. He danced with Mom. We all stood around them and laughed and clapped and cried. They have been through so much. I knew when I watched him that he had come alive again. My dad is back."

@

Like finishing one swing and preparing for the next, like holing out on three and then clearing the mind before teeing up on four, this transition to home required patience, letting go, and a readiness to start anew in each moment. This past month was filled with fluctuations—false starts and little victories—like birdies and bogeys. Now the questions were, "what has this round taught me? What have I learned? How have I grown?"

I struggled to embrace the fullness of these joys and sorrows. I eventually refused to reject any part of what this course handed to me. My question became, "How can I live a life with heart? How can I play my best game?"

With Dad home from the hospital, it was seductive to relax into the small view of "all is well." Fortunately, instead, an ongoing inquiry lived in me, "How can I live openheartedly?"

I found myself at my kitchen table, sipping my Energizing Tea for Women, contemplating, "How can I learn to let go daily, letting my heart break open?"

In moments of surprisingly deep gratitude for what felt like surviving a horrible round of golf, a disheartening day on the links, I now wanted to know, "How can I be in this life wholeheartedly?"

These were my queries. This was the work of the heart. As we had been shown, the future is promised to none of us; this moment is really all we have. In appreciation, I played with the paradox that a new aliveness was the biggest gift of Dad's brush with death.

Another question people frequently asked, "Do you have any advice for other families going through by-pass surgery?"

Maybe.

Of course, each emotional roller coaster ride is unique; each major golf tournament has its own long holes, tough lies and sand traps. Every golfer plays the links and the game differently. I could not imagine a right way for you. I am not even sure of the right way for us. I do know that through Dad's cardiac event, I learned to embrace the preciousness of life. Those few weeks blessed me with a wake up call. My prayer today is that I may stay awake. May I remember to be aware.

"Thought bubbles" came in my sleep. I scribbled them soon after opening my eyes. These daily notes arrived from some unknown source, and worked their way through my a.m. pen. I did not create them; I listened for them. During Dad's hospitalization, gentle nudges fell onto the paper. As I read these reminders today, they seem to have the quality of "Everything I Ever Learned I Learned from Dad's Open Heart Surgery," or maybe, "Golf Lessons from the Heart of a Champion." The following words may not make sense to you; they do not all make sense to me—I am learning to attend and, since the days of the frozen igloo, working to open the heart:

⑥ *Show up with a sharpened pencil. Pay attention.*
⑥ *It never rains on the golf course. But in life it drizzles and downpours. Plan accordingly.*
⑥ *Fore. Know where you are and know when to move out of the way.*
⑥ *Don't judge your performance. Accept everything as is, even spectacular wipe-outs, even landing in the rough. Whether you have a great day or a lousy day doesn't matter. What matters is that you step up to the tee, address the ball and play the game.*
⑥ *No matter what, always count your blessings.*
⑥ *Keep your eye on your own game. Stay right here, right now.*
⑥ *See into the distance. Sense the whole course.*

⑥ *Relax your swing. Move from your core.*
⑥ *The other person is not your opponent. The game is your challenge.*
⑥ *Prepare thoroughly. Trust your own pre-competition training to get you through.*
⑥ *Practice. Don't expect perfection. Practice more. Do your bucket work. Practice again.*
⑥ *Take one breath at a time. Tackle one shot at a time.*
⑥ *Visualize a positive result, then let go of expectations.*
⑥ *Slow everything down.*
⑥ *Get more comfortable with discomfort; develop increased tolerance for ambiguity. In this game, you never know. Anything can happen.*
⑥ *Nurture inner calm. Be sparing with your energy.*
⑥ *Stick to the fundamentals, let the last shot go, and let it happen.*
⑥ *Win humbly and be a winner when you lose.*

⑥

Do I have any advice?

Maybe.

My wish for you is the same as it is for us. May we look after the patient, and also look patiently within. While our loved one's physical pulse is being taken, may we learn to check our own emotional pulse. May we come to accept whatever feelings we find, remembering that *all* feelings are normal. May we then be better able to face what is asked of us. Finally, whatever our circumstances, whatever our experiences, and whatever our plan, may we interpret in the largest context possible the words of Bobby Jones,

> "To say that any round of golf offers a magnificent
> gamble in the way of form is to add nothing new.
> We all realize that we can never know in advance

how the shots will go on a particular afternoon. To go even further, we can have no assurance, after hitting seventeen fine tee shots, that the eighteenth will not be disgraceful. These are the uncertainties the golfer accepts as parts of the game, and indeed loves it all the more because of them."

THE NINETEENTH

SMELLING THE FLOWERS

While I owe much to golf, I think I've been able to follow Walter Hagen's advice: 'You're only here for a short visit. Don't hurry. Don't worry. Take time to stop and smell the roses along the way.'

Ray Lebel, at his induction
into the Maine Golf Hall of
Fame, 1993

Sunday, August 18, 2002

Rushed, I slammed the back door. I was late to join my husband, Jon, to make our reservations for brunch. The phone rang. I unlocked the door, pushed it open, grabbed the receiver within arm's length of the doorknob, and yelled to Jon, waiting in the car, "I'll be right there."

"Sue, it's Mom. What are you doing now?"

"I'm flying out the door. Why? What's going on?" I asked.

"It's about Dad. I thought maybe you could…"

My heart skipped, and I plopped into my kitchen chair to

listen. Not feeling much fear, I nevertheless wanted to pay close attention. "You thought maybe I could what?"

⑥

This was where Mom's phone conversation departed from the one I received three years earlier.

Mom explained, "Well, you know that Mark is playing the final round today of the Portland Club Championship. Vicki is caddying for him, did you know that? Dad is out there riding around in a cart doing rules."

"Dad didn't enter?"

"No, he decided not to compete this year. It's been so hot and he's not feeling very strong. He really hasn't played much this summer. He was afraid he might be too weak to play those two difficult days of golf with the tees way back and the course set up so long."

Since Dad played fewer tournaments and less golf generally these past three years, he had been busy on the New England PGA Rules Committee.

Mom continued, "John Boswell, the pro at the Club, called to tell me that today he is going to make a presentation to Dad after the final round ends. The Golf Committee decided to name the Club Championship Tournament after Dad—the Portland Country Club Ray Lebel Cup. Dad doesn't know anything about this. Boz knew he could get Dad to come to do rules, no questions asked.

Boz asked Dad if he would present the big silver bowl to the winner of the tournament. Dad is unaware that first there will be a ceremony to honor him for his years of golf, for his winnings, and for his years of service to the Club. The cup that Dad presents to the champion will have his name on it. I thought maybe you might want to come."

With this invitation, unlike the one three years before about whether or not to get his car after Dad's admission to Maine Medical Center, there was no foreboding in my decision. "Yes, I'll come. Jon'll come, too."

"Oh, by the way," Mom added, "Mark is in contention. He's had two good rounds and was one of the leaders going out today. Wouldn't it be great if Dad could present the cup to Mark? I've called all the kids. I think everyone'll be there. Mark is due to finish around one o'clock."

Enthusiasm spiked with worry, I wondered, *Is this a good idea—to surprise a seventy-nine-year-old man with a heart condition? Won't he suspect something when he sees us all?*

None of the thoughts took hold, however. Even as I sat, talking to Mom, I mentally flipped through my closet. "What do I have to wear to the Club?"

Dad taught us to keep the mind focused and steady; mine was taking off right now in very strange directions. "Will we all be in the pictures?"

Puzzled and questioning, I nevertheless applied sunscreen and found clean shorts. Today the Portland Country Club would honor my dad for his thirty-seven victories, for doing more for golf than any other player, and for giving so much back to the game.* Of course I'd be there.

6

It was a beautiful Maine summer afternoon: In the seventies, bright blue sky, and we were in sundresses or shorts and t-shirts. From where we relaxed on the plush fringe of the practice green, we could view the golfers coming up eighteen, the deep azure water of Casco Bay glistening behind the last three holes. Spectators gathered: some cigar-smoking golfers finishing their Sunday afternoon round; Al Noyes, Mike Franceour and Frank Langlois, golfing buddies; and employees of the pro shop. A crowd formed and we proudly spread the news. "As of today,

Later Ray Lebel was given an honorary life membership to PCC.

the Portland Country Club Championship will be called the Ray Lebel Cup."

"How wonderful. He deserves it. I didn't know that but I did know it was just a matter of time," we heard from the growing gallery.

"Yes, I know. That is as it should be," winked the old-timers. It had been hush-hush for months. The Golf Committee had hidden the trophy, as it was engraved, "The Ray Lebel Cup" since the decision almost a year ago.

Our family, golfers and non-golfers alike, stretched out on the grass. Jon played Gin Rummy in the shade with Sarah, Ann's daughter. Ann stood with Mom and me near the eighteenth green. "Where's Dad?" we kept asking.

"Out on the course somewhere," was the common reply.

Mike, his wife Suzi and their children Andy and Kaitlin sat in the Grill Room eating tuna salad, dill pickles and thick chips, waiting for the last golfers to finish. Paul, Dave and his wife Lisa and daughter, Lindsay, joined them, and Mark Koshliek, Vicki's husband, came to see if anyone wanted a "cold one."

Mark's family was there; his wife Donna, their daughter, Kailey and son, Mark Jr. They wanted to know, "Where's Mark?"

A young pro shop worker, keeping the score board, informed us that Mark was not playing well, and would likely not be able to fight his way back to the top.

Finally we spotted Dad, wide-brimmed straw hat with a thick band, dark blue golf shirt, sleeves a bit beyond the elbow, khaki Bermuda shorts, a bit below the knee, tiny white golf socks. We could not find his eyes behind his huge dark glasses, but his smile disclosed his delight in that Rules cart.

He spied us, all in a clump at the eighteenth green and laughed, "What is this? All my family is here."

I covered. "Mom told us Mark might come in low gross, so we wanted to cheer him in."

"Well, you can go home now," Dad signaled with a wave, "He's a few strokes back and a couple of the other competitors are hot today."

Inwardly we giggled. Outwardly we kept our secret. "All the more reason to stay. Mark'll need the support."

My stomach performed flips as I waited for the last group to come up eighteen. Once more I heard Dad wondering, "What the heck is my whole family doing here?"

After an hour, I spied Mark climbing the long uphill end of the eighteenth fairway. He was shaking his head, without the usual bounce in his step. Sweaty and slightly limping carrying Mark's clubs in the hot sun, Vicki dropped his bag to announce, "He'll probably finish at about ninety today."

Dad motioned for us to leave, but we had another reason ready. "Oh, let's stay just to see who wins."

At last the tournament ended. It was time for Dad to present the prize to the winner. The group of forty or so moved as a pack from the eighteenth green to the hardtop outside the pro shop, in front of the leader board. The clicking herd of cleats attracted more curious onlookers. Mark turned in his card and joined the spectators. Dad reached for the heavy silver bowl, about to introduce Jon Piper, a first time winner. Dad called him "Johnny, one of the young kids." Jonathan Piper is my age.

But John Boswell, the pro, stepped in and lifted the huge shiny trophy.

"Before we present the trophy to this year's winner," he began, "I have a few words to say."

Dad stepped back to listen to Boz, expecting him to say how

much Johnny had improved this summer, and what a good tournament this had been. Boz turned to Dad, faced him directly. "Ray," he started, "this trophy has had your name on it for so many years now that we decided your name should be engraved on it for good. From now on, this tournament will be called the Portland Country Club Ray Lebel Cup."

Dad's face turned ashen. Dazed, he fell against the gray clapboard pro shop behind him.

"Oh, my. Oh my goodness," he muttered.

I fixed my eyes on him still questioning of the wisdom of surprising him. He recovered quickly. He wiped his forehead with the palm of his right hand, and dabbed his face with the white handkerchief from his back pocket.

Boz now recited statistics of Dad's wins, his work for golf and the Club, his longevity in the game. His lovely words blurred together for me, faded into the wings, as I watched Dad center stage. Dad pointed at us as if to say, "NOW I see why you're all here."

He raised his eyebrows, opened his mouth, and thrust his tongue in wide-open surprise. Gathering himself enough to present the cup to Jon, each exchanged glowing remarks about the other. I did not hear them.

Shaking his hand, patting his shoulder, and embracing him, his friends all made presentations, too. Frank Langlois presented him with an extra-long driver to help with his shortened backswing. Frank mentioned, "Ray is the only person who could manage this seven-foot club." Everyone applauded and then someone said, "Go ahead and hit it, Ray."

He did. We all laughed as the ball shot down the fairway.

Al Noyes spoke incredulously of playing with Dad for the past thirty or so years without ever seeing him "lose his cool."

Mike Franceour stood next to Dad, now holding Frank's extended driver, put his hand on Dad's back and announced to the crowd, "Without a doubt, this guy has conducted himself in such a manner that it speaks volumes about his character both on and off the golf course. He is a gift to the game of golf, to the State of Maine and to the Portland Country Club."

Dad lost and regained composure again and again. He seemed overwhelmed, then smiled and finally offered words of thanks. Through my tears, I did not remember them.

⑥

Later that night, I called Dad to see how he was feeling. "Pleased," he reflected. Then he added, "You know, I had kinda lost interest in golf this year. I've done a little work in the shop with Dave and Mark, and I love my digital camera and the courses I've taken in computer photography. I still have my frame shop here, and there's a lot to do. I'm starting to see there's more to life than golf. Ever since my surgery, I'm just so happy to be on the green side of the grass that I can't get too excited any more about whether I miss a three-foot putt.

It's funny. I heard today that some people thought the new name for the tournament was to be 'The Ray Lebel Memorial Cup.' Well, even though my heart almost took me out a few years back, I'm still here. And even though I'm not playing much, my heart will always belong to golf. I've always loved that game. I learned pretty much everything I know through golf, and much of my success in life came from golf. It was really nice to be honored today to receive that trophy, but, you know, I didn't play all that golf and work that hard for the sport to get rewards. Golf has given me a lot in life and I think it's important to give back."

Three years after Dad's brush with mortality, I sometimes forgot its most poignant lesson for me; immortality is an illusion, a delusion. We are all going to die. Despite an important awakening, I found myself sleepwalking again and again. Having adopted a certain complacency, now I was reminded to make each moment full and precious.

❦

Now, we do not know from day to day what the future holds for Dad and his health. Every now and then I hear him say those words he so casually uttered a week before his routine checkup several years ago, "I'm a little worried about my cardiac status."

Sometimes he senses an arrhythmia, sometimes shortness of breath and unusual fatigue. Even though he may yet walk many fairways, life is uncertain. What is certain is that the wisdom my father learned on the links now teaches us moment-to present moment that, whether in golf or in life, it is important to give back.

Ray Lebel is a legend, a champion by all measures. And winners know that it is possible to live limited by vascular constriction, and still cultivate a heart as wide as the world. Giving credit to a fellow celebrated Maine golfer, Dad is quick to point out that Mark Plummer, of Augusta, is his present-day hero. Fame comes and goes. People have their moments in the spotlight, and then everything fades. Circumstances change. Only the lessons are timeless.

Dads are not supposed to get sick. But they do. In the end, all I can conclude is that we must, right here, right now, open our hearts in the midst of inevitable heartbreaks. I once thought Dad would live forever. Now I treasure every smile. Dad's following words spoken from the heart of a champion about the fickle nature of golf, ring through the ages and the unpredictability of the human condition. "You never know what can happen. It's a guessing game. That's just the way it is. And despite all the emotional ups and downs—or maybe because of them—if you love the game, you go out there and play anyway."

⑥

Printed in the United States
70969LV00002B/1-177